CLINICAL METHODS
IN COMMUNICATION DISORDERS

CLINICAL METHODS
IN COMMUNICATION DISORDERS

THIRD EDITION

William R. Leith

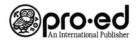
pro·ed
An International Publisher

8700 Shoal Creek Boulevard
Austin, Texas 78757-6897
800/897-3202 Fax 800/397-7633
www.proedinc.com

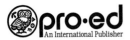
An International Publisher

© 1984, 1993, 2002 by PRO-ED, Inc.
8700 Shoal Creek Boulevard
Austin, Texas 78757-6897
800/897-3202   Fax 800/397-7633
www.proedinc.com

Library of Congress Cataloging-in-Publication Data

Leith, William, 1927–
    Clinical methods in communication disorders / William R. Leith.—3rd ed.
        p. ; cm.
    Includes bibliographical references and index.
    ISBN 0-89079-885-0
    1. Speech therapy.   2. Therapist and patient.   3. Communicative disorders—
Treatment.   I. Title.
    [DNLM: 1. Communication Disorders—therapy.   2. Language Therapy—methods.
    3. Speech Therapy—methods. WM 475 L533c 2002]
    RC423.L414   2002
    616.85'506—dc21

                                                                    2001048262

This book is designed in Goudy.

Printed in the United States of America

1 2 3 4 5 6 7 8 9 10   06 05 04 03 02

*This book is dedicated
to all the clinicians
in my chosen profession.*

CONTENTS

PREFACE

When I was introduced to the field of speech therapy in 1950, the emphasis was on therapy and did not vary much from the four basic types of disorders: articulation, voice, language, and stuttering. I studied with Dr. Charles Van Riper at the Western Michigan College of Education when the field was less than 20 years old. The American Speech-Language-Hearing Association (ASHA) did not yet exist, so we were part of the Speech Association of America. Our conventions were a part of the Speech Association, and it was rare to find a department offering a major in speech therapy. We were usually associated with departments of speech or English. The field was in its infancy, but the seeds of growth had been planted. Research and technology led the way for the ASHA to become an outstanding professional association. As I look back, it has been an awesome period of growth.

Our profession has made great strides during the approximately 70 years it has been in existence. We have researched deeply into the etiologies of the various disorders; we have devised numerous diagnostic instruments; we have studied carefully the speech and language process. However, there seems to be one crucial facet of our profession that has escaped our attention: the therapeutic process itself. We have been so preoccupied with studying the disorders that we have paid scant attention to the process through which the disorders are premeditated. From our research and empirical base, we know what new speech behaviors to introduce to our clients, but the *how* of therapy remains a mystical procedure. We learn the *how* of therapy by observing other clinicians and through our own experiences in the clinic room. To say the least, it is not a well-understood process. Perhaps, because of the vagueness of the process, we have very little insight into the most frustrating of all clinical problems: achieving carryover of new speech behaviors into the client's natural speaking environments.

The history of any profession functions primarily to familiarize its members with past accomplishments and failures. Having this information, future generations of the profession can embark from this point of professional development and not repeat all of the trials and errors their predecessors made. As I attempted to share my clinical history with my students so they would not repeat my clinical trials and errors, I discovered that I had neither the vocabulary nor the clinical concepts necessary for this sharing. I found myself limited to sharing anecdotal clinical experiences, hoping that the students would learn, at least by rote, how to deal with specific clinical situations.

As I became more frustrated with this problem, I began to study therapeutic procedures carefully in an attempt to find a vehicle through which I could share my clinical history. I found answers in cognitive–behavioral therapy and various principles of learning. By combining these factors, I developed a theoretical framework, which I refer to as the Clinical Interaction Model (CIM). This theoretical framework provides both the vocabulary and the concepts that allow me to share my clinical history with my students. I can explain, according to specific principles, what has transpired in a clinical interaction. cognitive–behavioral therapy and the CIM are the focus of this book.

This book is about therapy—not what new speech behaviors are to be introduced to the various types of clients we work with, but rather how these new speech behaviors are taught. I am not proposing a new therapy approach. I will be discussing the same therapy that good clinicians have been practicing for years. However, the CIM is a way to view therapy so the clinical interaction can be understood as a predictable teaching/learning exchange between the clinician and the client.

Therapy is not a mystical procedure. It is a learning situation that is based on learning principles that govern the interaction between the clinician and the client. Once the principles are understood, therapeutic interaction becomes a lawful process that can be planned, and its outcome can be predicted. The main purpose of this book is to set forth those principles that govern our clinical interactions. This information should provide the clinician not only with the necessary means of planning a logical treatment program, but also the insight necessary to solve procedural problems if a treatment program is not yielding the desired results.

It is my sincerest wish that the information included in this book will be of value to you, the reader. My students and I have found that the CIM increases the efficiency and the effectiveness of our therapy. The core of our profession is the practicing clinician providing clinical services to those who have communication disorders. Our professional reputations rest directly on the efficiency and effectiveness of these services. I hope the concept of the CIM will have a positive influence on your clinical services.

As you read the book, pay particular attention to Chapter 3, Cognitive–Behavioral Therapy: A Model. The ground rules of therapy are presented and discussed here, including all of the pertinent learning theories and concepts. Motivation, one of the most important factors in therapy, is the focus of Chapter 4. The learning environment and all of its implications are the topics discussed in Chapter 5. These three chapters form the basis for therapy based on solid clinical principles.

The last chapter is a departure from the general tone of the book. Whereas the book is more general in nature, not focusing on any specific disorder, this chapter deals specifically with stuttering. I added it when I discovered to my dismay that cognitive–behavioral therapy was missing from the literature on stuttering.

A book of this nature is dependent on the input of many people, and I would like to thank them for their assistance. I would first of all like to thank Dr. Mary Jane Dettman, who guided me on the original idea for the book and consulted with me during all of the revision. I also greatly appreciate the guidance I received from Dr. Greg Mahr from Ford Hospital, a psychiatrist, a clinical partner, and a fellow researcher, as I wrote the chapter on counseling.

A word of thanks to Dr. Alex Johnson, head of the Department of Audiology and Speech–Language Pathology at Wayne State University in Detroit, Michigan, for his most timely suggestions regarding Chapter 13. I also want to thank Dr. Kenneth St. Louis (one of my earliest students) at the University of West Virginia for his candid recommendations on Chapter 13. A very special thanks is given to Kristine Sbaschnig, the Clinical Coordinator in the Department of Audiology and Speech Sciences at Wayne State University. She has helped me in many ways throughout the years. I would also like to give special thanks to Betty Fusilier from the University of Central Arkansas for her invaluable help in revising this edition and for her unique assistance over the years, including introducing me to the outstanding catfish dinner at the "Gas Station/General Store/Restaurant" in Toad Suck, Arkansas (Yes, Virginia, there is a Toad Suck, Arkansas).

LIST OF FIGURES

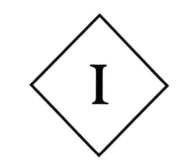

THE FOUNDATIONS OF THERAPY

CHAPTER

1

FUNDAMENTAL CONCEPTS

◆ Synopsis

Compared to other professions, ours is still in its infancy. Indeed, like young children, we often ask, "Where did we come from?" We also sometimes question exactly what we do and how we do it. This chapter addresses these questions and calls your attention to the basic issues concerning the services that the speech–language pathologist provides.

You are about to read a unique book. Essentially, this book concerns the application of learning theory and a communications model, and the interaction between the clinician and the client. The learning theory and model form the base of a teaching/learning interaction we call *therapy*.

Clinical Methods in Communication Disorders is not a documented research reference book. It is a practical orientation to communications between clinicians, clients, and others involved in the treatment program. This book is not concerned with what new behaviors to introduce in response to various types of communication disorders (it is assumed that you received this information in specialized courses), but rather with how to teach these new behaviors to the client. This book is not concerned with how to plan therapy, but rather with how to view therapy so it can be planned. *Clinical Methods* is not concerned with various ancillary procedures involved in therapy, such as writing lesson plans, selecting diagnostic tests, and writing reports, but focuses on the actual therapy process of teaching new behaviors or concepts to clients. This book is not a detailed procedural book on how to take case histories, how to conduct interviews, or how to do a diagnostic evaluation or other procedures. Rather, it presents a way to approach these procedures to increase their efficiency and effectiveness.

This book is a theoretical approach to the clinician–client interaction we call *therapy*. The theory and accompanying models provide you with a way to view therapeutic interactions so they are no longer reflexive and extemporaneous, but are seen as practical applications of laws of learning. Along with the practical elements of the theory and models, this book provides a vocabulary that allows you to think in broad, clinical concepts as you plan appropriate therapy. The theory and models also provide the tools for solving clinical problems. Think of this book as a practical guide to good therapy planning and application.

Before going any further, let us establish a more personal form of communication than that usually found in textbooks. I, the author, am writing this book for you, the reader, in an attempt to share with you my thoughts regarding the treatment of communicative disorders. The informal style of the book was requested by numerous clinicians whom I consulted. I trust that the informal, conversational style and the incorporation of some humor will not distract you from the pertinence of the information I am trying to convey. For the sake of brevity and clarity, I will refer to the speech clinician as "she" and the client as "he" for the remainder of the book.

If you are a practicing clinician, I hope we can relate on a professional level and share our experiences. If you are a student, I hope you find my thoughts and experiences helpful as you pursue your training as a speech–language pathologist. I am not attempting to set forth new clinical approaches in this book. Rather, I want to share with you the *Clinical Process* concept, which I feel will explain in a clear and concise manner what we do in our treatment programs and why we do it. The Clinical Process is an overview of the treatment program and consists of a number of interrelated clinical processes. We will be establishing a new vocabulary related to treatment so we can communicate clinical concepts rather than only describe clinical behaviors. If we have a clearer understanding of the treatment process and the concepts that are involved, we will be able to plan more effective therapy and resolve clinical problems faster and more easily.

Who Are We and What Do We Do?

The first question we should ask ourselves as speech–language pathologists is "Who are we?" We represent a professional group whose purpose is to remediate or correct communication problems. These problems are in the general classifications of articulation, voice, language, and rhythm disorders. We are a legitimate profession with a research base from which we draw information concerning the etiology and treatment of the various types of disorders with which we work. We have a well-established professional organization and numerous training programs that adhere to professional standards set forth by our national organization. We test and certify our professional people and have established ethical standards that govern our professional behavior. One of the main problems we have faced over the years is what to call ourselves.

Perhaps the problem of professional identification was best put forth by one of the leaders in our field who, in addressing our professional standards, wrote:

> In reviewing these problems, it became apparent to me that not only are our training standards vague, but we have never really come to grips with the problem of defining the nature of clinical work. Before long we shall have to decide just what the professional fields of clinical speech and audiology are. Perhaps this statement seems a bit naive, but do we really know our rightful boundaries? What terms describe us: Teachers? Clinicians? Therapists? Technicians? Counselors? It was surprising to me to realize that aside from an occasional brief discussion in textbooks, our literature contains little which defines explicitly the scope of our profession. (Bloomer, p. 11)

It might surprise you to realize that this was written in 1956. In fact, this same problem exists in our field today; we are still not sure what the scope of our profession is or what term to use as a professional title.

In the early years of the profession, we referred to ourselves as *speech correctionists*, but this term came into disfavor and a search was begun for another label. The title *speech therapist* was then coined. This term continues to be used but is not accepted by all members of the profession because of semantic problems with the word *therapy*. The term has some medical overtones, inferring that therapy can only be performed with medical prescription or supervision. Although this may have been the case a number of years ago, it no longer applies. For example, the occupational therapist provides many therapeutic services without medical prescription or supervision.

The most common and probably most preferred professional title currently used to describe us is *speech–language pathologist*. If we interpret this title literally, we find the title still does not accurately describe all of our professional activities. The term *pathology* relates more specifically to the study of diseases and their manifestations. We do study disorders of the communication system and we do diagnose the communication disorders in our clients. So if we stretch a point, perhaps we do function as speech–language pathologists during our evaluations of our clients. However, this is only a small part of our total professional activities. Once we have diagnosed the particular problem, we then provide some sort of service to remediate, eliminate, or reduce the problem. Those clinical services constitute the majority of our professional time, and we should acknowledge this in our professional title.

I would like to use the terms *speech clinician* and *clinician* to describe us in this book. I have not overlooked the area of language disorders, but for brevity's sake, I will use the shorter version. As long as we all understand what the terms infer, we should have no communication disorder. And, obviously, this is important in a book about communication disorders.

I would like to take this semantic problem one step further. I am not suggesting we change the professional title we have settled on, but I want to make a point regarding the type of service we provide. I would suggest that the term *teaching* accurately describes what we do with our clients in therapy. What do we actually do in interactions with our clients? We teach! Let us view teaching as the creation of new behaviors, new concepts, or new information in a client. We do this either *directly*, by presenting the new behavior, new concept, or new belief to the client, or we do it *indirectly*, by manipulating the clinical environment so that the new behavior, new concept, or new belief evolves from the environment.

Now if we are teaching, we would indeed hope that the client is learning. This would appear to be the true test of our therapy: "Is the client learning what we are attempting to teach?" If we extend this concept, we would then ask the question, "Is the client learning what is expected within a reasonable period of time?" We are confronted, then, with two questions regarding our therapy: "How *effective* is it and how efficient is it?" I truly believe that these are separate questions.

Let us consider an example that will illustrate the difference between effective and efficient therapy. The client we will discuss is a 5-year-old who has an [s/l/r] problem. The therapy used with the child was effective in that all sounds were corrected and they were produced correctly in all positions and all social contexts. The only problem with the therapy was that the client was retired and on social security before therapy was completed. Yes, the therapy was effective but it certainly was not efficient. We should ask ourselves about the effectiveness and efficiency of our own therapy.

Several factors influence the effectiveness and efficiency of our therapy. Some we can control, but others we can only adapt to since they are dictated by the agency or clinic where we are employed. An example of the factors we must adapt to would be how often we meet with and how much time we spend with the client. This has a direct bearing on the efficiency and effectiveness of our therapy. However, if our therapy plan is, itself, ineffective, seeing the client more often and for longer periods of time will not help. We also need to consider the client's motivation. This will be one of the main themes of this book, so we will not get deeply involved in it at this time. Other factors include how many clients are seen at one time, the homogeneity of the group, the cognitive level of the client, and so forth. Regardless of these factors, as professionals we are accountable for both the effectiveness and the efficiency of our therapy.

How Do We Learn To Do What We Do?

Our professional learning starts in our training program. We enter a program to learn to be a speech clinician. In order to function effectively as a clinician, we must have three things: (1) the ability to establish rapport with our clients, (2) the technical knowledge associated with the various communication disorders, and (3) insight into teaching strategies so our clients can learn what we are trying to teach them. Let us discuss each of these clinical prerequisites.

What is rapport? This is extremely difficult to define, but perhaps we can describe it. Basically, it means there is mutual respect between the clinician and the client. For a more in-depth review of the concept of rapport, see Chapter 2 in Othmer and Othmer (1989). Rapport is also related to the attitude of the clinician toward therapy. If the clinician enjoys both the therapy process and the client, this attitude is reflected in the therapy; it is enjoyable to both parties. The client then respects and enjoys the clinician. Where does this attitude come from? A key word seems to be enthusiasm. We all have observed boring therapy where the clinician has no enthusiasm. We cannot deal further with this issue since we have yet to learn how to instill enthusiasm in a clinician. Let us hope that people enter the field because they enjoy it, and that enjoyment is the seed of enthusiasm.

As for the technical knowledge, we take specialized courses in the various disorders, where we learn the etiological theories of the disorders, descriptions of the disorders, evaluative procedures, and what new behaviors, concepts, or information we need to teach the client in order to minimize or eliminate the problem. Our training seems to cover the technical information quite well.

How many times have student clinicians complained that all they got out of a class on a particular disorder was theory, nothing practical? What do they mean by *practical*? They learned how to evaluate the disorder and what new behaviors to introduce. They were introduced to the various etiological factors that might influence their treatment. They became intimately familiar with all aspects of a particular disorder. This information is all "practical." Therapy is impossible without it. But their complaints are still justified in that such classes give no practical information on how to do therapy.

Learning How To Do Therapy

Where do we learn the *how* of therapy—how to actually *do* therapy? We learn from our clinical observations, our course in clinical methods, our clinical experiences, and our conferences with our clinical supervisors. Clinical observations are usually assigned to students early in their training program, primarily so they can get a general idea of the speech clinician's role in the clinic room. Additional observation assignments maybe made later in training to study the clinical interaction in therapy.

It is probably during these observations that student clinicians begin to seek *recipes* for treating the various types of disorders. Since the students do not understand the therapy process at this point in their training, they attempt to formulate a standard approach to each disorder based on what they have observed.

The material covered in clinical-methods courses or their equivalents varies widely. In some courses, the *how* of therapy is discussed and perhaps even demonstrated. The problem instructors face in presenting the *how* of therapy is the lack of published material on this aspect of therapy. (This book was written to help fill this gap.) In any event, the students do gain some insight into the therapy process in these classes as they prepare for their forthcoming clinical experience.

We now move into the third and fourth factors, clinical experience and conferences with a supervisor. It is at this time that a clinical team is formed—the student clinician and her clinical supervisor. After a client is assigned to the student and the client's files have been reviewed, the clinical team has a conference to plan the therapy. Lesson plans are written and reviewed. The supervisor's main job at this time is to get the clinician to give up the recipes and actually plan a unique therapy program for the individual client. This effort continues even after the clinician has started therapy with the client. Planning is difficult since the clinician has no experience to draw on, only the information gained in observations, the clinical-methods course, and the first few conferences with the supervisor. Recipes offer security blankets for floundering clinicians.

The conferences with the supervisor focus on evaluating the therapy that has been completed, planning where the therapy will go in the future, and solving any clinical problems that have arisen. Unfortunately, the evaluation of the therapy is after-the-fact: The mistakes have already been made. At first, these conferences are somewhat limited in their effectiveness because the clinician's clinical vocabulary and grasp of clinical concepts is limited. The vocabulary is important since a clinician cannot explain clinical concepts if she does not have an adequate clinical vocabulary and, conversely, she cannot understand concepts if she does not understand the terms being used in an explanation.

The clinician sometimes has great difficulty in catching on to what the supervisor is trying to teach. However, as the clinician gains clinical experience, the conference becomes more effective since the clinician is learning clinical concepts and a more extensive clinical vocabulary. As this happens, the supervisor gradually introduces indirect teaching (teaching by manipulating the conference so that important clinical concepts and principles are discovered by the clinician). The supervisor leads the clinician to the answers but does not provide them. As the clinician gains insights into the clinical process, the supervisor provides less guidance and the clinician begins to operate with more independence. One of the important clinical tools taught in this way is problem solving. The clinician cannot operate independently until she has mastered her strategies of solving clinical problems.

Eventually, the student clinician completes the requirements of the training program and, upon graduation, is ready to function professionally as a speech clinician. We now move into another phase of learning the *how* of therapy through clinical experience: on-the-job training.

Let us look at this positively. A good clinician never stops learning to do therapy. There are always new types of clients, new challenges, new approaches. It is impossible for a training program to prepare the student for every possible type of client and clinical setting. We simply leave one learning environment and enter another. Let us hope we made all our serious clinical errors during our training, while we were under the guidance of our clinical supervisor.

In earlier eras of our profession, training programs had not developed the extensive supervisory skills that are found in training programs today. They took many years to evolve. Clinicians who were trained in the 1950s and 1960s did not have the supervision opportunities available in today's training programs. At that time, clinical skills were learned through trial and error, with little opportunity to consult with a supervisor.

The clinical history of our field (the record of our professional advances in providing clinical services, the result of development of new strategies and techniques, and the acquisition new knowledge about disorder types) is extremely important. The historian in our profession is the clinical supervisor, and history is important so that we can avoid repeating the errors of previous generations of clinicians. The idea is to learn from others' mistakes. This is the challenge of supervision: to keep the new clinician moving ahead, avoiding a repeat of others' errors. If our profession is to continue making clinical progress, new generations of clinicians need to begin where previous generations left off, and not start again at the beginning. It makes no sense to repeat all of a previous generation's clinical errors. And yet, in training students to do therapy, it seems like that is exactly what is happening in our profession.

Perhaps if I shared some of my own clinical training experiences with you, you would have a greater appreciation of the value of our clinical history. My clinical training took place many years ago; however, I am certain you will find many similarities in our individual experiences. Our profession has not made a lot of progress in teaching the *how* of therapy over the years.

I started my training by observing other students in my program doing therapy. These student clinicians were one or two years ahead of me, and many of them were working with their first client. I observed very carefully and made notes on what I thought was transpiring. The only persons I had with whom to discuss my observations were the student clinician and other student observers. What was I attempting to learn through my observations? I supposedly had much of the technical information, but I needed to understand the teaching strategies used by the student clinician. My conferences with the student clinician were what is commonly referred to as "the blind leading the blind."

After relatively few hours of observation of other students doing therapy, the moment of truth arrived. I was enrolled in a clinical practicum course and, shortly thereafter, received notification that I had been assigned a client! Following the initial combination of thrill and total panic, I went to the clinical files and reviewed what the previous clinicians had written. My client's file was extremely thick with report after report from student clinicians the client had trained. These were the truly frightening clients since, after training so many generations of student clinicians, they knew more about the therapy than the student clinicians. Having reviewed the client's file, I then discussed my new client with those other poor souls who were attempting to get their courage up to meet their first client. Misery loves company.

Following a brief conference with my clinical supervisor, I wrote up my first, but definitely not my last, clinical lesson plan. How I struggled with that first attempt to figure out what to do for an entire therapy period! I tried to plan what I would say to the client the first time we met. What would I say to his parents? How would I establish that mysterious thing—rapport—that everyone talked about but could not explain? Would I like my client? Would my client like me? This is when I learned the real meaning of anxiety.

My first client's name was Gary. He was a 9-year-old, language-retarded, hyperactive, destructive child. In our first meeting, I called upon my vast reserve of observational experience (about 30 hours) and found, much to my chagrin, that my observations did not include a client of this nature. Undaunted, I plunged ahead with the clinical activities I had so carefully prepared in my lesson plan. As you might suspect, the first 30-minute clinical meeting was a total disaster. I ignored Gary and he ignored me. I was so preoccupied with following my lesson plan that I was oblivious to the fact that Gary was paying attention to everything in the therapy room except me. My lesson plan and my therapy were very efficient; I finished the entire therapy plan in 15 minutes. I will not go into the morbid details of how the remaining 15 minutes were spent. The only bright side to this clinical experience was that, in the future, my therapy could only improve. As I look back, I hope that Gary eventually learned as much from me as I did from him. I also hope he survived the multitudes of clinicians he trained. My clinical supervisor attempted to point out all the things that were wrong in the therapy session, but there was just too much to cover. She struggled through this client with me, but most of the time I did not understand the points she was attempting to make. I did not have either the clinical vocabulary or the clinical concepts needed to fully appreciate the guidance she was trying to give me. Furthermore, these conferences were few and far between and always occurred after I had already made the mistakes.

In retrospect, I think I knew what I wanted to teach Gary, but I did not understand the clinical process. I did not know *how* to teach him. I only knew what I had seen. I did not understand the procedure, but I could imitate it if all the conditions from my observations were the same in my therapy. Realistically, this just does not happen. Every client is different, as are the interactions between clients and clinicians. My first clinical experience could be used as a classical example of how *not* to do therapy. If there was anything I could have done wrong that I did not do wrong, it was simply an oversight on my part. I repeated every clinical error ever made by any clinician in the entire history of our profession.

The value of clinical observations early in my training program was quite limited. Yes, I saw things going on that I could repeat in another clinical situation, but this was imitation of a process. Competent clinical planning could not occur since I did not understand the process itself. This type of learning is akin to learning brain surgery by observing a second-year medical student perform a delicate operation on the brain without receiving background in neuroanatomy or neurophysiology. Before I observed ongoing therapy, I should have been made aware of the basic principles that are involved so I could have understood what I was seeing. It also would have been nice to see a trained, professional clinician demonstrate therapy.

Therapy Should Be Lawful, Not Awful

In my years as a teacher, clinician, and supervisor, I have seen many examples of "awful" therapy. Before we describe awful therapy, let us apply the *OP Rule*: Awful therapy is always done by *Other People*. Awful therapy is boring; both the clinician and the client are bored. There is no rapport between the clinician and the client. The therapy is not planned, it is not organized, and there is little interaction between the clinician and the client. Neither the clinician nor the client is aware of the clinical goal, and the therapy has no purpose. Even the clinical activities have no purpose since there is no goal. Everything appears to be occurring randomly. Obviously this list could go on and on, but I will let you fill in other factors from your own observations.

Therapy involves both the teaching skills of the clinician and the learning skills of the client. In order to develop teaching skills, the clinician must understand *how* and *why* people learn. With this information, teaching strategies can be developed that are both effective and efficient. The interaction between the clinician and the client should not be a random learning experience. It should be guided by specific principles and laws of learning. If these basic principles and laws are understood and used in clinical planning, the clinical process becomes a predictable interaction with a predictable outcome. Also, if a teaching strategy is planned according to these principles and laws but (due to an unforeseen factor) the procedure is not effective, the principles and laws will indicate where the problem is and how it may be resolved. Problem solving is one of the most important things the clinician is called upon to do.

This is our professional challenge—to be able to plan an appropriate and effective clinical program for our clients, regardless of the type of communicative disorder manifested, and to make sure that the program is efficient. This is a professional obligation as well as a moral obligation. Our first task to increase our clinical efficiency is to organize therapy into a logical sequence of events.

The Treatment Sequence

As we move into the treatment of communication disorders, let us consider what the steps of our treatment program are. In our discussion, the four steps of treatment will be:

1. Evaluation and planning. Our first task is to determine if the client actually has a communication disorder and, if so, its type and severity. Thus, the initial step in the treatment sequence is the diagnostic evaluation. If a communication disorder exists, we need to determine the reason it exists, since this will influence the type of treatment program we are going to plan for the client. We must also be concerned with the cognitive functioning level and the communication skills of the client, since these factors have direct bearing on how we will approach teaching new behaviors.

After gathering data, we decide on the classification of the disorder and plan a treatment program. The type and severity of the disorder, the presence of any organic factors, and the client's cognitive level and communication skills are all considered when determining the behavior-change goal and planning the general approach to treatment.

Our findings and recommendations are all brought together in the final conference. We explain to the client and significant others our classification of the communication disorder, its severity (if pertinent), and the treatment program we feel is appropriate for the client. When the conference is completed, therapy begins.

2. Getting the new behavior to occur. Having decided what behavior to focus on and what the behavior-change goal is, we then proceed to teach the new behavior. Learning theory is the base of our interactions with the client. We employ specific strategies that are designed to teach the client to produce the new behavior.

3. Habituating the new behavior. Once the new behavior has been performed, it must be habituated in the clinical environment. The new behavior must occur correctly and without prompts or cues from the clinician. It must be stable in the clinic room before it can be generalized to the client's natural speaking environments.

4. Generalizing the new behavior. Therapy is not complete until the new behavior is occurring spontaneously in all of the client's speaking environments. The speech clinician is involved in this last step of therapy, though her clinical activities will change. She is no longer working on the speech in the clinic room. Clinical activities during this phase focus on helping the client perform the new speech behavior outside the clinical environment.

It is in this step of therapy where we sometimes must deal with new behaviors that do not habituate. They reduce the severity of the disorder but since they do not habituate or generalize, their effectiveness is limited; the disorder continues to exist. The most obvious example of this concerns our therapy with clients who stutter. Behaviors (such as rate control, which, according to some proponents, eliminates stuttering) cannot be habituated to the point where they occur reflexively and consistently in all speaking situations. We must create maintenance programs for clients who stutter, programs that enable them to maintain a much reduced level of severity.

During my early years as a speech clinician, I felt the most secure in the first step of the treatment program. As members of this profession, we have established reliable and valid evaluative procedures for all the communicative disorders. I would include here *diagnostic treatment*, where the final decision regarding diagnosis of the communicative disorder comes only after some treatment has occurred. I was also comfortable determining the behavior-change goals and planning therapy for my clients. This information was included in the courses I took in my training program, and I could also get the information from almost any pertinent textbook.

I felt much less secure with the second step of treatment—the therapy phase. I knew many techniques, such as the stimulus method, motokinesthetics, providing models, and so forth. However, I did not understand the dynamics involved, and I did not have a regular supervisor to go to for help. It was difficult discussing this aspect of therapy with other clinicians, since we did not have a vocabulary to describe what was transpiring in therapy. This was the *how* of therapy, and I had to learn it through trial and error. Later on, I found that this was also the part of the treatment program that I could not teach my students; thus, they could not avoid repeating many of my clinical errors.

The third step—habituation—did not present insurmountable problems. With drill work and conversation, I was able to get new behaviors to occur consistently and correctly in the clinic room. I may not have been very efficient, but I always managed to stabilize the behavior in the clinical environment.

I felt very insecure with the fourth step of the treatment program— generalization. From my discussions with other clinicians, I found that I was not alone in my insecurity. It appeared that this was the major problem that most clinicians faced. And this is the step in the treatment program that has been discussed least in our literature. We were able to create the new speech behaviors in the clinic room successfully, but had difficulty in getting the new behavior out the clinic room door. It seemed to disappear in the hall on the way back to the waiting room. And with some clients, especially stutterers, we could never get the new behavior to habituate or generalize. When I was new in the profession, this last step in treatment was the most challenging and was suspect both in terms of effectiveness and efficiency. This seems to be the same clinical problem plaguing the profession today: We are least effective and efficient when it comes to carryover.

The Clinical Process

The core of this book is the *clinical process*. It focuses on the direct clinical interaction between the clinician and the client, and it addresses the teaching and learning processes that form the foundation of therapy. The clinical process consists of the four steps in the treatment sequence and provides us with an overview of the complete treatment procedure.

Finally, regardless of how well we are prepared for therapy, we must consider the effects of certain laws of nature on the clinical process. We cannot prevent their occurrence, but if we understand them we can minimize their effects. After much deliberation and study, I have set forth these laws, which can be found in Appendix A. I would recommend that you study them before proceeding with this book.

CHAPTER

2

THE OUTSTANDING CLINICIAN

◆ Synopsis

To be outstanding, the clinician needs to perform a number of specific behaviors and activities. One list of such behaviors comes from an article written by a speech pathologist who suffered a severe stroke. Another list was prepared by several clinical supervisors. Then there are those skills that are displayed by all outstanding clinicians. The synthesis of all this is the Clinical Behavioral Profile, which evaluates both positive and negative characteristics of the individual clinician.

What Makes a Great Clinician?
Ask the Client

In 1973, one of my former students, Joysa (Joy) Post, who had obtained both her bachelor's and master's degrees in speech–language pathology and who had worked successfully in the field for several years, had a serious cerebral vascular accident (CVA) at 29 years of age. Following the CVA, Joy spent almost a year and a half totally nonverbal, with no means of communication. Because her cognitive functions were unimpaired and due to her professional training,

Joy was extremely frustrated with both her inability to communicate and the treatment procedures to which she was subjected. She was finally taught to communicate through eye blinks, which she used to indicate the appropriate letters to spell words. This was a tedious process, but at least she could communicate. This situation continued for another year and a half.

Then very suddenly, in 1976, Joy was able to speak. She spoke in complete sentences and with essentially normal speech. It was a startling event that appears to have been precipitated by some factor during a surgical procedure. No one has been able to explain the recovery of her speech, even though her medical records were examined by medical teams. It happened instantaneously, as she explained in an article she wrote (Post, 1983).

The spontaneous recovery of her speech occurred 3 years after her CVA. This is not to say that her speech was totally normal following the recovery, but the single remaining problem was a dysarthria that affected the articulatory production. In the ensuing years, she has continued to improve her communication skills by reducing the effects of the dysarthria.

During this time, Joy had been professionally evaluating both her emotional responses to her condition and the treatment programs provided by the speech–language pathologists who worked with her. With her professional background, she was aware of what the clinicians were or were not doing, and she formed some very strong opinions about how speech–language pathologists should work with clients with her type of problem. She wrote her story and presented it at the Metro Speech and Hearing Association meeting in Denver in the fall of 1981. Many people attending the meeting suggested that she share her insights with others in the profession by publishing her story. She sent me a copy of the paper and, after reading her account, I also urged her to publish it. Joy's story, which follows, is in her own words.

At Joy's request, I edited the paper, but the editing was limited to focusing the paper on the most pertinent point and organizing the material sequentially. Although Joy's condition may be unique and her comments not applicable to all clients with a severe language deficit, I feel there is a message in this story for all speech–language pathologists.

I'D RATHER TELL A STORY THAN BE ONE
By Joysa Post with William R. Leith

I'm going to relate a unique personal experience. It is unique both because of my age and because I am a trained speech–language pathologist with a master's degree. My experience began on Memorial Day 1973. I was with my parents at their cabin in the Rocky Mountains about 50 miles west of Fort Collins, Colorado. I was sitting at the table writing a term paper when I had an uncontrollable sneeze which seemed to trigger a massive CVA. My neurosurgeon diagnosed it as a congenital malformation at the base of the right cerebellum characterized as VonHippel syndrome. It is a rare condition and even more unusual when one survives it.

Within a matter of minutes my life changed completely. I was rushed to the nearest hospital which was in Fort Collins, 50 miles away on winding mountain roads. I was in surgery seven hours during which part of the right lobe of the cerebellum was removed, leaving me completely paralyzed. While I was in intensive care for 21 days, I had to have a shunt, had a cardiac problem, was on a respirator, and had to have a tracheotomy. I was nonverbal for three years and unable to eat for four years as I could not chew, suck, or swallow. Most things that people take for granted were very difficult for me like crying, smiling, laughing, coughing, shrugging my shoulders. In fact, any type of movement was extremely difficult and most were impossible. On June 18, 1973, I was moved to the Rehabilitation Unit of Boulder Memorial Hospital in Boulder, Colorado.

What was my initial speech therapy like? My speech–language pathologist would write a correct response on the chalkboard. I would watch to see how she made it and look at the correct response. My vision was blurred and sometimes I saw double so my responses were not always accurate. Nursery rhymes were read to me. On these, the speech–language pathologist would read the rhyme leaving out the last word on the line, then had the missing word on a card. By holding a card in each hand and telling me what was on each card again, I was to look at the correct word. I remember one instance when the rhyme was "Hickory, Dickory, Dock." One card had "dock" and the other had "tock" but my vision was not good enough to discriminate between the "d" and the "t" and I didn't look at the correct response even though I knew what it was. A number would be omitted from a written sequence, like 1, 2, 4, 5, and I was to figure out what was missing. Words were printed in two spellings and I was to tell which one was correct. The only way I was able to respond early in therapy was by moving my eyes. For months, my clinician had me smelling and feeling things. Many things were done that were not very stimulating or interesting. When I became bored, which was often, I would pretend to be asleep!

Early in my therapy, my speech–language pathologist tried to use a language board with me which required my pushing a control button. After months of practice I could finally move my thumb. I could never use the language board because it was very frustrating. I was supposed to use my thumb to push the button until I came to the correct letter to spell a word. My reaction time was so delayed that I could not do this. I could not release my thumb from the control fast enough, so many times I would pass the letter I wanted and then could not reverse the control and get back to the correct letter. At the end of 16 months in hospitals where I had intensive physical, occupational, and speech therapy, I still had no means of communication and the only voluntary movement I had was to move my right thumb and blink my eyes.

It was very evident that I was nonverbal but not until 16 months after the onset was any kind of communication system devised that I could use. I was extremely frustrated because I could understand everything but could not respond. Since I could not talk, people talked louder to me or talked as if I were a little child. The first comment to me by most visitors was "Do you remember me?" Of course I did!

In September 1974, I was moved into my parents home in Sterling, Colorado. All of my clinical services were provided in the home. After 16 months of being totally unable to communicate, I had a great clinician who devised a language system which I could use! I could finally communicate with people! Let me explain how it worked.

I would close my eyes while my clinician would say the letters of the alphabet. When she came to the letter I wanted I would open my eyes. This was difficult since my reaction time was very slow, and sometimes I would open my eyes too soon, while other times it came too late. My speech–language pathologist was very patient and together we might complete one sentence during an hour of therapy. With much practice, I became more accurate at opening my eyes on the letter I wanted. The communication methods I used were in sequences as follows:

1. *Word spelling.* Just as I have described it. Opening my eyes for the correct letter I wanted.

2. *Yes/No.* Everything had to be phrased to me as a question with a "yes" or "no" answer. I kept my eyes closed for "no" and opened wide for "yes."

3. *Use of parts of speech to construct sentences.* I again would open my eyes for the part of speech I wanted but still had to spell nouns and verbs. This method was faster because of sentence patterns. Not everyone could do this with me as they had forgotten the parts of speech.

4. *Head nods.* I finally got control of my head and could give a quick nod. This was faster than eye blinks and more accurate.

5. *Division of the alphabet into three sections and the use of fingers.* The alphabet was divided into sections A-G, H-Q, and R-Z. After I was able to move my fingers, I would signal one finger for the first section, two fingers for the second, and three for the third. The person would then say those letters and I would give a head nod for the correct one. I

could use this method with everyone; I had paper handy for them, but I had to remember everything I was trying to spell.

During this time, my speech–language pathologist and I were working on breathing exercises and vocalizing. Many techniques were used to help me breathe so I could talk, but the most effective for me was simply an ice cube run across my diaphragm. A book was placed on my abdomen and by watching it move, I could tell if I was breathing correctly. I could say about 20 words by the end of May 1976. On June 10 of that year, I had to go to Denver for surgery on my Achilles tendons. This was three years and two weeks after the accident. I had the surgery on my tendons at Presbyterian Hospital in Denver, Colorado. Three days after the surgery, *I SPONTANEOUSLY BEGAN TALKING*. I could say everything! Without going through steps, I could talk in complete sentences. On an articulation test I gave myself, I found substitutions, omissions, and distortions. I also determined that my voice quality was harsh with some hypernasality. I also spoke in a monotone. After my inability to talk for three years, all of these errors were insignificant. I also found that I had developed a tongue thrust. When I was awake at night I would practice my exercises for it and within six weeks that problem was alleviated.

Chewing, sucking, and swallowing exercises were very important for me to make my tongue functional. Without use, my tongue had become thick and flat, the 't' was not pointed, and I had no control of the tongue while eating. After the accident, I could not swallow any kind of liquid or food so surgery had been performed and a gastrostomy tube inserted so I could be fed a formula. I gradually learned to eat soft foods and the exercises were a great help.

My speech is still improving. Some times I talk too loud. I still do a lot of talking on residual air. I try to drop my voice at the end of a sentence, put on word endings, try not to omit letters or substitute sounds, and remember to breathe after a phrase. So many of these things that people take for granted, I must think about each one. I know what I should be doing, but there are times when I don't accomplish my goals. It is not because I do not want to, but sometimes I simply can't. This is a very important factor that all clinicians must recognize. With clients, like me, some days we can do things but the next day we cannot do them.

At first it was very difficult for me to accept my condition. To know I was once *normal* and now I could not even do what a baby does automatically was very frustrating. I could not even shed a tear, but I cried a lot inwardly. My mind was clear and I knew exactly what I wanted to say but the words just would not come out. I understood what the clinicians wanted me to do, but I just could not do it. I know that they were frustrated with me, but they did not seem to understand that I was also frustrated with me. There were so many things I wanted to tell the clinicians about my needs and how they were doing therapy, but I could not get the words to come out. Many times over the years I could have given up but I was surrounded by people, including some of my speech–language pathologists, who gave me encouragement and support. Because progress was very slow, and at times it seemed there was none, many of my clinicians wanted to quit, but my family and I would not let them give up with me.

Being in a wheelchair, I learned that if I accept my condition others would also. A good sense of humor has helped. Having patient and cheerful people visit is good therapy because I knew my friends were pulling for me. It is important for a person to know that they are not alone. What hurt me most was that some of my good friends stayed away. I guess they could not handle my condition, were afraid, or thought I was worse than I was. Actually, I am not different, I just do many things differently. If I can accept my mode of transportation, my speech, and my many handicaps but others cannot, then they are the handicapped, not me.

One of the hardest things for me to accept was that I could not do even the simplest task. Things I had done for years were extremely difficult or impossible. It was hard to be so dependent when I had been so independent. I never thought anything like this would happen to me. When I graduated from college the thought of being in a wheelchair was the furthest thing from my mind. Since the accident, I have great empathy for all handicaps. Does the average speech–language pathologist have the same empathy? Let me shed some light on this.

I feel the most important trait of a good clinician is a genuine caring and patient attitude. If one has a lot of "textbook learning" and little empathy for the client, progress will be limited. One speech–language pathologist I had gave me the feeling that when she saw me she thought, "Well, here's Joy again. What shall I have her try today?" Needless to say, I made very little progress with this clinician. She was never really prepared for therapy, and I knew she was just putting some things together on the spot to keep me "busy." I knew that her knowledge of my condition was severely limited. I think a client without my background would have recognized this also. I did not get a feeling of professional or personal concern or even professional competency from this clinician. I needed a clinician who cared and was interested in me as a person, a clinician who could make me feel secure her knowledge of my problem.

Clinicians should not try and "fake" therapy. Several of my clinicians did this and I knew it. Even if I was not a speech–language pathologist, I would have known it. Why didn't these clinicians admit that they did not know all about my condition and ask for help? How much of my life did they waste by faking their therapy?

The speech–language pathologist is an extremely important person to a patient who cannot communicate. You put all of your faith in this person who represents the profession that is going to help you learn to talk again. I remember one clinician I had who came to my home to provide therapy, and she would come in her bib overalls. It was hard to have faith in a person who dressed so casually. In my mind she viewed me and my problem just as casually. I wanted my clinicians to dress professionally, even if it was a white coat.

Another thing that has a big effect on the attitude of the client is enthusiasm. All speech–language pathologists need to be more enthused about their clients, to greet clients as if they were glad to see them, and to have a positive attitude about the clients. When I was depressed and the clinician was really not interested in me, I became even more depressed. It was wonderful when I would do therapy and the clinician was cheerful and friendly. Knowing that the clinician cared would bring me out of my depression.

If I am patient with myself in trying to reach my goals, the therapist must also be patient. When a clinician was impatient with me it would make me angry with her and then I would not work in therapy. I had taken years to learn some of the things a clinician might ask me to do. And she would be impatient if I took an extra second to do it! Remember, some days I can do something but other days I cannot.

It was nice to have a clinician who had a sense of humor and who made therapy interesting and fun. I still had my humor but several of my speech–language pathologists had lost theirs. Their therapy was boring and so were they. I was never motivated to go for therapy with these clinicians.

Therapy should be meaningful and have a purpose. As an adult client, my clinicians could have explained the purpose of their therapy and made it clear to me what they expected me to do. Many times I was confused as to what they wanted of me and why. Their therapy should have been directed toward my needs. I was a prisoner in my own body wanting to express my inner feelings. Listening to rhymes and smelling things was not meaningful to me and it did not have a purpose.

Finally, I want to mention dignity. Even though I was totally nonverbal and unable to move anything but my thumb, I still wanted to be treated as an adult, not as a child or as though I were retarded. I could still think clearly and I was insulted when a clinician treated me as less than an adult.

I am a perfect example that long-range goals are a necessity. It has taken me eight years to get where I am. On October 15, 1974, 1 eye blinked this message, letter by letter, in a diary my clinician kept for me, "If I could change the situation, I would speak and write my feelings to everyone." Now, almost eight years later, I am doing exactly that. I hope that you learned something from my story. Many clinicians just do not realize how much clients like me depend on them for moral support as well as professional treatment. We want you to care about us as well as care for us.

The following section was written by Joy in January 2001. She was asked to review the original article, which was published in the second edition of this book, and then respond to what she had written. There were no revisions or corrections made in her comments.

"As I reread my article I wrote about 20 years ago, I realize my life has gone through various stages: denial, anger, frustration and now acceptance. My health has been restored. I am able to be in a wheelchair all day, which was a major accomplishment because at first sitting in it for 2 hours was the maximum. At first I wore gloves, as my hands were too tender to push my chair. When the original surgery was done the neck muscles were cut so holding my head erect in the chair was most difficult. My first wheelchair has a headrest. My balance was the one thing that has not returned. I have done extensive water therapy and can walk in the water due to the fact that the water would hold me up. I walked in the water with very little support from my therapist. Since I could not swim before, everything from breathing, diving, walking was nothing short of a miracle. While doing water therapy I devised several pieces of equipment that I could use to help my balance as well as several other patients.

I have been at home since September 1976. My parents remodeled our home to make it accommodating for me. At first, we had a hospital situation here. Equipment involved was a hospital bed, a Hoyer Lift, wheel-in shower, etc. Not only was a positive attitude from me needed but my parents needed a lot of patience and understanding. Teamwork was essential. Now, the hospital setting is not needed. I was fortunate when I had a CVA that my intellectual capabilities were not impaired.

I have gone to Northeastern Junior College where I took computer classes. I am now able to work in a first grade class. I have volunteered daily for the past 15 years. In 1988 I was given an award by the South Platte Education Association as "Friend of Education." I am sure it was a motivation factor to be able to work with children again.

I have been very active in my church, serving as a Deacon, an Elder, and on various committees. I have spoken to many groups and although my speech is still distorted, at least I am verbal.

I am able to do most things now even though the things I accomplish are slower and done differently."

When I first read Joysa's story, I was overwhelmed with her incredible tale. I was very impressed with her evaluation of the clinical services she had received. For many years, I had the students in my clinical courses read her story to get some appreciation of the client's view of therapy and the clinician. As I reexamined the story for inclusion in this book, I made a list of those behaviors Joysa felt (both as a speech–language pathologist and a person with a severe communication disorder) were important for good therapy (see Table 2.1). We could not ask for a more highly qualified person than Joysa to comment on behaviors that separate the outstanding clinician from the average one.

One of the most basic ingredients in any interpersonal relationship is *humanness*. Without this, relationships are sterile and impersonal. If we remove humanness from therapy we might as well have a computer maintain all contacts with clients and turn therapy into a purely mechanical interaction. Nothing can replace the humanness in therapy, although the human interactions might be supplemented by computer programs or other types of mechanical or electronic devices.

Table 2.1
Qualities Important in Speech–Language Pathologists

Humanness

1. Caring for the client as a person
2. Having patience with the client
3. Being empathic to the client and his or her problems
4. Giving the client moral support
5. Maintaining a positive attitude
6. Treating the client with dignity

Professionalism

1. Making long-term plans for therapy
2. Being prepared for therapy
3. Demonstrating professional competency
4. Appearing in professional dress
5. Maintaining a meaning and purpose for therapy
6. Keeping the goals of therapy clear

Humor/Cheerfulness

1. Having enthusiasm for the therapy
2. Being cheerful in front of the client
3. Having a sense of humor in therapy
4. Making therapy enjoyable for the client

One of the common problems we must deal with is our tendency to "talk down" to clients with severe disabilities like Joy. They often seem so helpless that we speak to them as we would a young child; we ignore their concerns and thoughts. When we do this, we rob them of their dignity. We need to understand their plight, to identify with their struggle to survive, to appreciate their frustration, to tolerate their impatience with themselves and with us. We need to be caring clinicians. When we consider these factors, we can better understand why Joy feels that humanness and caring are essential behaviors for an outstanding clinician.

Professionalism cannot be underestimated for its impact on therapy. Professionalism does not mean adopting a superior attitude or being haughty to clients. It simply means behaving in a way that inspires the client to have confidence and respect in the clinician. If the client does not have faith in the clinician, minimal clinical progress will be made. Humanness and professionalism not only mix well, they are essential for good therapy.

With regard to humor, a wise man once said, "Don't take life so seriously; you'll never get through it alive." Many people in our profession take themselves too seriously, failing to see any humor in anything about their profession or even themselves. This lack of humor seems to be highly correlated with the number of letters in the professional degrees people have. It also seems to vary according to the severity of the disorder being treated, with less humor displayed with serious disorders and more humor with mild disorders. And, of course, with less humor there are fewer smiles. Perhaps there is a feeling that in dealing with serious handicaps we need to look serious and act seriously, and this means not smiling, looking stern, and removing any traces of cheerfulness. Is there a possibility we have this backward? As Joy pointed out, she needed some humor to help her deal with her serious problems. Unfortunately, this was not always forthcoming from her clinicians. A smile is a wonderful clinical tool for maintaining morale and motivation.

Which behaviors from Joy's story and in Table 2.1 are most important? Perhaps we should first get your opinion. Rank order the behaviors in each category, with the most important number first and so forth. Once you have your ranking, we can check it against the opinion of an expert. I sent the list of behaviors to Joy and asked her to rank the behaviors in terms of what she considers the most important. Her ranking of the behaviors is as follows:

Humanness: 1, 6, 2, 3, 5, 4

Professionalism: 2, 3, 4, 5, 6, 1

Humor/cheerfulness: 1, 4, 2, 3

What Makes a Great Clinician? Ask the Supervisor

Supervisors also have opinions about what behaviors contribute to a clinician's being outstanding. This issue is discussed in depth in the *Handbook of Supervision: A Cognitive Behavioral System* (Leith, McNiece, & Fusilier, 1989, Chapter 6), a companion book that extends the themes of this book into the area of supervision. Good therapy is dependent on a good clinician, and to be a good clinician the individual must satisfactorily perform 43 behaviors listed in Table 2.2. Naturally, the beginning clinician cannot perform all the behaviors at a satisfactory level. That is why there is clinical training—so the beginning clinician can learn to perform the behaviors. These 43 behaviors are listed in Table 2.2 according to their categories. Their operational definitions can be found in Appendix B. The list in Table 2.2, makes you realize that outstanding clinicians must work hard to achieve their level of proficiency. Good therapy is a demanding activity both for the client and the clinician.

Table 2.2
Important Behaviors for Clinicians

Planning

- Formulates long-term goals
- Formulates objectives session-by-session
- Modifies the clinical program when change is indicated
- Chooses materials appropriate for the client
- Has a rationale for clinical procedures
- Structures plan for maximum number of responses
- Demonstrates progress to the client
- Includes significant others in therapy plan

Interactions: Clinical and Supervisory

- Demonstrates sensitivity and awareness
- Relates to the client as a person
- Maintains awareness of affect in therapy
- Removes negative, personal factors from therapy
- Demonstrates initiative and independence
- Projects a positive image in the clinical setting
- Responds positively to supervision
- Keeps client/significant others informed regarding clinical status
- Interacts positively with other professionals

(continues)

Table 2.2 *Continued.*

Management

- Keeps accurate records
- Uses stimulus control in therapy
- Manages client behavior
- Maintains client motivation and attention

Procedures

- Makes clinical goals clear to the client
- Maintains goal-oriented therapy
- Appropriately uses teaching materials and activities
- Selects appropriate instructional techniques
- Teaches client to differentiate incorrect from correct behaviors
- Uses time-efficient procedures
- Demonstrates clinical flexibility
- Uses modeling, information, guidance, and feedback in therapy
- Uses rewards and penalties in therapy
- Teaches the client self-evaluation
- Maintains appropriate client talking/response time
- Develops appropriate client behavioral data-collection system
- Maintains focus on session goals

Diagnosis

- Administers tests accurately
- Demonstrates appropriate clinical observational skills
- Makes appropriate test interpretations and recommendations
- Writes professional reports

Additional Clinical Responsibilities

- Observes rules of the clinic
- Prepares for clinical conferences
- Contributes alternative procedures in clinical conferences
- Produces professional AR written work
- Develops self-supervision skills

Special Skills of Good Clinicians

Before getting into this section of the chapter, we should define what we mean by a *skill*. A skill is a special talent that we perform well. When we talk about a person being a skilled pianist we mean he or she has a special talent (playing the piano) and does it very well. A person may have some talent for playing the piano for sing-alongs and still have no skill as a pianist. Skill is something we do that is outstanding.

All of the behaviors mentioned so far are dependent on the clinician having certain skills. If the clinician does not have the necessary skills, the behaviors cannot be performed adequately. The skills we will discuss here fall into three categories: perceptual skills, cognitive skills, and performance skills. These skills make clinical interactions possible, since the interactions are based on receiving information, thinking about the information, and reacting to the information. As shown in Figure 2.1, information originates from the evaluation, conferences, and therapy. The information is received through specific perceptual skills, processed through a variety of cognitive skills, and then reacted to through specific performance skills. These performance skills are reflected in therapy, in conferences, or with written and oral reports. Let us consider each skill as it relates to clinical performance.

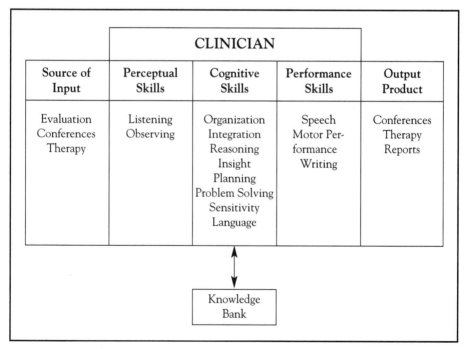

Figure 2.1. Skills related to clinical competency. Clinical competency is dependent upon perception of the incoming information, dealing cognitively with the information, and basing performance on the outcome of the cognitions. During cognitive processing, the clinician relies on her professional knowledge to assist in decision making.

Perceptual Skills

Listening. Listening skills are vital to good therapy. During history taking, conferences, and counseling, the clinician must listen carefully to what the client, significant other, or other professional is saying. This form of data collection is also vital to clinical progress. In counseling, particularly, the clinician must not only listen to the obvious verbal information but also must attempt to discern subtle messages and agendas, both verbal and nonverbal.

During therapy, the clinician must not only hear what the client is saying but also how he is saying it. She must be involved in both the content and the context. Exacting judgments are necessary to differentiate between correct responses and *almost* correct responses. AR clinical progress is dependent on these listening judgments.

Observing. Observational skills are essential in the context of evaluating behavioral performance to make certain they are physiologically and anatomically correct. I once supervised a blind clinician who was teaching a child to produce the [f] sound. Acoustically the sound was perfect, but, unknown to the clinician, the child was producing it with the lower teeth in contact with the upper lip.

Observational skills are also important in observing nonverbal communication in counseling and conferences. Facial expressions, eye movements, gestures, and posture are all important in forming opinions about the meaning of the verbal information being passed and the attitudes and beliefs of the person giving the information.

Cognitive Skills

Organization. Perhaps the most important cognitive skill is organization, because it is the most basic cognitive skill related to planning and problem solving, which comprise the core of good therapy. Organization consists of the ability to arrange seemingly unrelated bits of information into meaningful, sequential relationships. Once the information is organized, the event or situation that yielded the information is much easier to comprehend.

Integration. Integration is the ability to take the organized information and combine it into larger, integrated information units. The information is then no longer only sequential; it is integrated into thematic or topical databases. The original information base is now more gestalt in nature.

Reasoning. Reasoning allows the individual to reach conclusions or inferences from the sequenced or integrated databases. All databases are now meaningful units and the source of further consolidation.

Insight. Insight is that special skill that allows us to perceive the true nature of an event or a situation. This is usually done through intuition—a feeling of knowing and understanding that is independent of any reasoning but that may draw upon the databases.

Planning. When a person has the skill of planning, he or she is able to integrate solutions to problems into therapy plans. This means they can plan for both short-term and long-term goals, and their teaching strategies are appropriate for the client.

Problem Solving. Problem solving is a form of insight learning. It enables us to resolve problems by comparing the known facts of the problem with related themes or topic databases. When the solution is reached, it comes suddenly as the relationships between the variables and the pertinent information from the databases come quickly into focus. The solution is often accompanied by the person uttering such words as "Oh, yeah!" or "Aha" or even a lightbulb flashing on top of the person's head.

Sensitivity. When a person is sensitive, he or she is aware of and responds appropriately to the needs and feelings of others. This is the source of empathy toward clients and their disorders. This skill is directly related to the perceptual skills of listening and observing.

Language. Language skills consist of both the necessary vocabulary and the syntactical skills to clearly explain thoughts, ideas, and concepts to a variety of listeners whose communication skills range from basic to very advanced.

Performance Skills

Speech. Speech is, perhaps, the most important performance skill. It is the vehicle that makes almost all clinical activities possible. Through speech, we are able to have conferences with clients and significant others, perform evaluations, perform therapy, communicate with clients on nontherapeutic levels, consult with other professionals, and so forth. Speech skills are essentially based on cognitive language skills, vocabulary, and syntax. However, the end result, speech, is a motor performance. Speech must be clear and intelligible to all listeners.

There is also the act of projecting speech so it can be heard. The clinician must not mumble so the listener cannot hear her. She must speak up in a professional manner. There is also the context that prosody (melody, rhythm, and accent) adds. We indicate questions, statements of fact, and other contexts through the use of rising and falling slides and variations of the two. People who do not use prosody while they speak are very boring, hard to listen to, and difficult to understand. This communication disorder is most commonly found in the lectures of many professors who shall be nameless but can be identified by all readers.

Motor Performance. By motor performance, I mean the clinician must be able to demonstrate how to make sounds both auditorily and visually. If speech motor skills are lacking, the speech production will demonstrate an articulation disorder or some other substandard performance. One of the most important clinical tools we have is modeling. And most of the time we use modeling to combine acoustic production with physiological production. To show the client how to make the sound, we open our mouth and let them see the positions of the articulators. As they look in, they also hear the production of the sound. This gets very tricky with sounds like the [r]. When you open your mouth wide to let the client see how you are producing it, the sound is distorted into something unidentifiable. If the child learns this new sound, therapy has to start all over again to correct the newly learned but unidentifiable sound. This presents a serious problem since, in all probability, the clinician will again attempt to teach the [r] by opening her mouth and letting the client look at the positioning. Again, another unidentifiable sound is learned. Hypothetically, this therapy routine could go on forever.

Writing. There are several writing levels of which the clinician should be aware. First, there is *professional* writing as seen in professional journals. The secret to this style of writing is to make the sentence so convoluted and the terminology so jargonish that no one clearly understands what is written, even the author. In a mistaken way, our profession seems to feel that the more difficult something is to read, the more it reflects higher levels of intelligence and professionalism. I have always been confused by this. Ours is a profession that deals with communication disorders, and yet we set up a standard that flies in the face of intelligent writing. Anyone who has ever tried to read a journal article knows what I mean. Unfortunately, this writing style has also crept into many of the books in the profession. I have decided that this writing style is a reflection of people who cannot write, writing to other people who cannot write.

Second, there is a form of writing that says what you want to say in the shortest and clearest form possible. In most instances, "big" words are unnecessary and only confound the reader. The purpose of writing is to communicate (share) concepts, ideas, thoughts, or conclusions. Why confuse the communication with bad writing? When writing, use the KISS rule: Keep It Simple, Stupid. Impress your reader with your knowledge and information, not with your ability to complicate your writing to the point of its being unintelligible. And let us not, under the guise of professional communications, demonstrate idiosyncratic priggery by foisting off on readers tomes filled with jargon and arcane terms for the singular purpose of intimidating the victimized reader with our charade of intellectual prowess and professionalism, while prostituting the purpose of all written documents, that is, to convey information gleaned from our life experiences to another individual in the most succinct and explicit form possible. Or, put another way, don't write to try to impress people but to clearly share information, and beware of run-on sentences—longer and more complicated does not mean better!

Special Attributes of Good Clinicians

Common Sense

How does one define *common sense?* It is native intelligence, the ability of a person to sense the obvious and act accordingly. The old saying, "He doesn't have enough common sense to come in out of the rain," says it all. All the behaviors and skills discussed earlier are of no use if the clinician does not have common sense. Common sense would dictate, for example, that if a child was running and screaming around the therapy room, therapy would have to wait until the child was brought back under control. Or if the child is brought to therapy when ill, the child will not be able to perform up to capacity and allowances must be made in therapy that day for the illness. Common sense dictates what should be done in most therapy situations. Whether or not the clinician listens to her common sense and responds accordingly is another matter.

This point was best made by Watterson (1988) in his cartoon *Calvin and Hobbes.* Calvin's mother is scolding him for breaking a dish and asks him how he did it. Calvin replies that he was carrying too much and dropped it. His mother then explains that his problem is he doesn't have any common sense. Calvin protests loudly, saying that he has a lot of common sense. In the last frame he qualifies his protest, saying he just chooses to ignore his common sense. Let us hope that Calvin does not decide to enter our field when, and if, he grows up.

Positive Personality

Personality is the visible combination of the individual's physical, mental, social, and emotional characteristics. It is greatly influenced by the individual's attitudes, feelings, and beliefs. Each person's personality is a reflection of who they really are. It is that part of each of us that other people see and relate to.

For purposes of our discussion, let us consider two basic types of personality in terms of interactions with others. First we have the withdrawn personality. We often refer to these people as shy. They do not enter into conversations easily and usually only respond to others, rather than initiate conversations. People with withdrawn personalities might have some difficulty functioning as clinicians since they are essentially followers, rather than leaders, in social interactions. However, many clinicians who are withdrawn are able to adjust to new situations and become much more outgoing than they were during their initial contact with the client.

The second type of personality, the outgoing personality, manifests itself in a person acting assertively rather than shyly. People with outgoing personalities initiate conversation and interactions and are usually seen as leaders rather than followers. These people are easy to relate to and have an initial advantage as clinicians since they establish rapport rapidly.

Ability to Work with Others

The clinician must be able to work on a team with other professionals. This calls for openness and objectivity on the part of the clinician and on the part of other professionals including but not limited to classroom teachers, psychologists, occupational and physical therapists, and physicians. Sometimes, clinical conflicts arise among team members as to who "owns" what part of a client. For example, the speech therapist might say that it is her mouth and that occupational and physical therapists should stick with their parts, the arms and legs. Or, when a client needs to learn eating skills, there might be a territorial battle between the speech therapist and the occupational therapist. The ability to work with others is a skill that all members of a team must have. In essence, this means each team member must respect the professional skills and contributions of the other members of the team. A pediatric neurologist in Chicago, in his lectures on team rehabilitation of neurologically impaired children, used to say that there were enough STs, PTs, and OTs but not enough SPOTS.

The Clinical Behavior Profile

Now let us try to put this all together. We know what makes a good clinician, but how do we rate this combination of clinical skills and behaviors? The Clinical Behavior Profile (see Figure 2.2) is an attempt to pull all of this together into a clinical profile so we can get an overview of a clinician's skill levels.

I would like you to use the Clinical Behavior Profile to rate four clinicians. The first three will be clinicians you know and have observed. Be careful about showing them your judgments. They could be interpreted as "constructive criticism," and we all know that this is a term used to try to cover up pure and simple criticism. Call it what you will, it is still criticism, and this is hard to tolerate, especially from a peer.

After you have practiced by rating three other clinicians, it is time to rate the best of the clinicians you know, yourself. Be honest and see how you compare to the other clinicians you rated. This should be a lesson in humility. Keep improving your profile and trying to become an outstanding clinician.

TRAIT	NEUTRAL	TRAIT
Introvert		Extrovert
Passive		Aggressive
Impersonal		Personal
Insensitive		Sensitive
Reactor		Proactor
Impatient		Patient
Unsupportive		Supportive
Humorless		Humorous
Glum		Cheerful
Negative		Positive

Figure 2.2. Clinical Behavior Profile. The behaviors listed on the profile represent the best and the worst traits of a clinician. Using three other clinicians and then yourself, place a mark on the continuum between the extremes which you feel best describes that trait as it exists in the person you are evaluating. Compare your profile with the profiles of other clinicians.

COGNITIVE–BEHAVIORAL THERAPY: A MODEL

◆ Synopsis

Having established that our contacts with clients should be a teaching/learning experience, we need to understand the dynamics of the clinical situation. Our clinical interactions are governed by principles and concepts. If we understand them and carefully incorporate them into our therapy, our therapy becomes more effective and more efficient. This predictable and lawful interaction can be manipulated by the clinician in many ways to adjust it to the demands of each unique situation. This chapter concerns the Clinical Interaction Model (CIM) *that sets forth the operational aspects of this clinical interaction. This model will assist the clinician in planning therapy and resolving clinical problems when they arise.*

The Core of Therapy

Now that we know who we are and basically what we do, let us talk about the *how* of what we do. Essentially, we teach the client new speech behaviors, attitudes, or beliefs. The effectiveness of our therapy is dependent on how well the client learns what we are attempting to teach. The most important ingredient of our therapy is the client's learning. How does the client learn? There are many theories and concepts regarding human learning, but no single one satisfactorily explains all of the learning that goes on in the clinical environment. We cannot go into a detailed presentation of each and every learning theory or concept, but we will briefly discuss some of the basic assumptions and concepts of those theories that are of particular interest to speech clinicians. Since we are limited to a brief discussion, I highly recommend that you do additional reading in this area. The more information you have about the various theories and concepts, the better you will understand your therapy. I would refer you to the References and Further Reading section of this text. Because some of these references are quite theoretical and abstract, I suggest you start with *Psychological Theories of Human Learning* by Lefrancois (1972). I hope you can find the book, because he presents learning theory, which is notoriously dry and boring material, in a very humorous manner that makes for easy reading and good retention. I also recommend the books by Hegde (1985), Cornett and Chabon (1988), and Mower and Case (1982), all of which deal with therapeutic processes and procedures. Now, let us take a brief look at some of the more common learning theories and concepts that are used by the speech clinician.

Learning Theories and Concepts

Classical Conditioning

In classical conditioning, responses are elicited by stimuli. If the stimulus is not present, the conditioned response will not occur. In the conditioning process, a bond is established between the stimulus and the response so that each time the stimulus is presented, the response occurs. The name we all associate with this form of conditioning is Pavlov. Pavlov conditioned a dog to salivate (response) when a bell was rung (stimulus). This concept is clearly demonstrated by the Wizard in Figure 3.1. The dog has been conditioned to associate the ringing of a bell with food. So when the bell rings, the dog drools and slurps. The jester? Same principle? Exactly!

A treatment method has been devised that is related to classical conditioning—Systematic Desensitization. If a client has been conditioned to respond to a stimulus with fear, anxiety, and tension, he is taught an alternative response—relaxation. The stimulus is then presented in graduated steps, starting with the presentation of the least disturbing aspect of the stimulus. The process continues as the client maintains his relaxation until the client can remain relaxed even

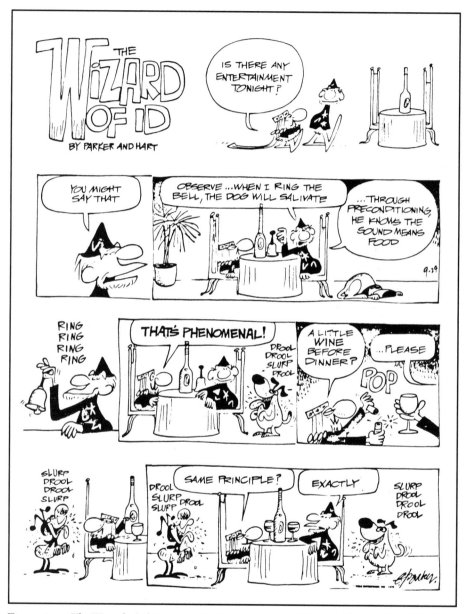

Figure 3.1. *The Wizard of Id.* Reprinted with permission of Johnny Hart and Creators Syndicate, Inc.

when the stimulus is presented at full strength. Clinical application of systematic desensitization is found primarily in the treatment of phobias that inconvenience a person. The procedure can also be used with stutterers who have fear of talking on the telephone. When the stutterer is relaxed and fluent, the telephone is gradually presented as the stutterer maintains his relaxation and fluency. If the stutterer tenses and begins to stutter, the hierarchy (look at it, touch it, pick it up) is temporarily halted until the stutterer regains his relaxation. The presentation then resumes until tension is present again. The procedure is continued until the stutterer is desensitized to the telephone. Many universities have desensitization programs to assist students who have uncontrollable anxiety associated with tests (my students highly recommended such programs).

Operant Conditioning

With regard to operant or instrumental conditioning, the response is not directly related to a stimulus. The response is emitted rather than elicited. Also, the learning experience is dependent on the consequence of the response. If the consequence is positive for the person, the response has been reinforced and the probability that it will occur again is increased. If the consequence is negative, the response has been punished and the probability of future occurrence is decreased. In Figure 3.2 you will see that Ziggy is learning to respond through reinforcement.

Chances are that when Ziggy goes back into the dog trainer's office he will fetch the ashtray because this behavior was reinforced. Will he also hand the dog trainer $20 each time he enters the office? This will depend on how much he likes Doggie Yum Yums.

As was just mentioned, we also learn things through punishment. It is a bit different in that, when our behavior is punished, we tend not to perform it again in order to avoid the punishment. This is a strong form of learning, as you will see in Figure 3.3.

Will Farley drink out of the toilet again? Not if he can help it. He will avoid this because he knows that when he does it, he gets banged on the head. Farley may be a dog, but he is not stupid. This is called learning the hard way.

The clinical applications of operant conditioning are found in all aspects of treatment of general behavioral disorders. Some programs are based on reinforcing appropriate behaviors, some on punishing inappropriate behaviors, and others use a combination of reinforcement and punishment. This clinical approach is widely used by speech clinicians in all forms of therapy. We encourage correct speech behaviors to occur through reinforcement and discourage incorrect speech behaviors through punishment. There are other theories of learning that

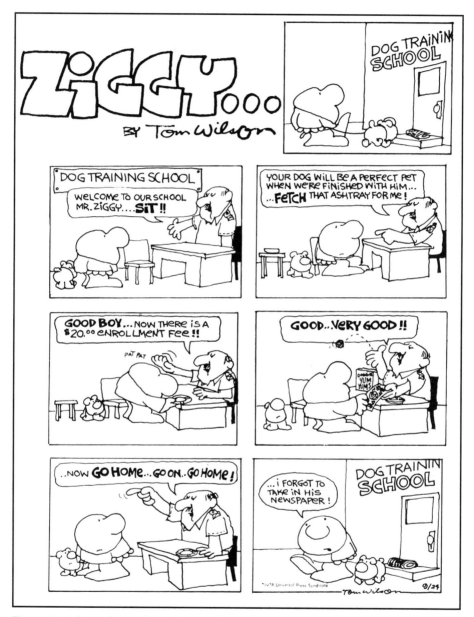

Figure 3.2. *Ziggy.* Copyright by Ziggy and Friends, Inc. Dist. by Universal Press Syndicate. Reprinted with permission. All rights reserved.

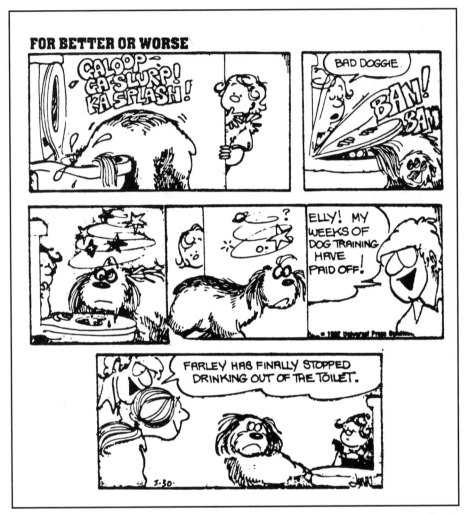

Figure 3.3. *For Better or Worse.* Copyright by Lynn Johnston Prod., Inc. Reprinted with permission of Universal Press Syndicate. All rights reserved.

are applied in the clinical setting but the operant approach is the one most commonly used by speech clinicians.

Modeling

One of the most common ways of learning to perform a new behavior is by watching and/or listening to someone perform the behavior and then attempting to reproduce the behavior. According to Bandura (1969), this is referred to as *modeling, imitation, observational learning, identification, copying, vicarious learning, social facilitation, contagion,* or *role playing.* We will use the term *modeling* for this form of learning.

Consider such activities as driving a car, swimming, or operating a computer. These could all be learned by trial and error or learned in gradual steps (shaping), but these forms of learning would not be very efficient. Think of what would have happened if you had learned to drive a car strictly by trial and error. Can you imagine the costs repairing not only your car but all of the cars you damaged? By the time you learned to drive you would not have been able to buy insurance, and the local police would have barred you from the streets. Learning to drive would have been more effective if you had had a model you could have used as a pattern for your own behavior (it is always better if the model is not provided by the parents of the beginning driver since this usually results in negative emotions and even worse language). When a model is presented, the learner has the goal behavior clearly set forth, and the randomness of the behavioral performance is greatly reduced. With a model, most behavioral performances are goal oriented.

It is important to recognize that many modeling–learning approaches assume that there is a reward associated with the performance of the imitated behavior. This reward could be either a direct reward for behavioral performance or the intrinsic reward of successfully imitating the model. We will assume this view of learning is through modeling.

Modeling is an important factor in understanding how children learn to talk. It explains why children learn to speak with the same accent or dialect as their parents. Speech clinicians have used this form of learning from the very beginning of the profession, and it is reflected in one clinician who tells her clients to "listen and watch, think about it, and then try it." We set forth the speech goal for the client by modeling it so the client not only knows what is expected of him, but he also has seen and/or heard it performed and has a better idea of how to recreate it.

Motor Learning

Motor skills are frequently referred to as perceptual–motor skills. This terminology is used to emphasize the coordination between the sensory input (perception) and the performance of the behavior (motor skill). The concept of motor-skill learning is typically applied to eye/hand coordination skills such as handling a tennis racket or swinging a golf club. In most references you will find that speech–motor learning is excluded from the category of perceptual–motor-skill learning and included as part of verbal learning. However, the concepts involved in perceptual–motor-skill learning are directly applicable to our therapy.

This is a complex form of learning and concerns the learning of specific motor skills. First of all, we need to define a "skill." Generally, it refers to a chain or sequence of motor responses (muscular movements) that are learned through the coordination of various sensory and motor systems in the body. The skill is then organized into complex response patterns. When we apply these principles to learning the motor movements involved in speech, the primary sensory systems that are involved in this learning experience are the visual and auditory systems. An example of the application of this learning system to speech is learning a consonant/vowel/consonant (CVC) syllable by listening to and watching a person produce it. The CVC syllable represents a sequence of muscular movements involving several motor systems (tongue, jaw, lips). This CVC syllable is then organized into a complex response pattern—the client's speech.

Let us consider the sequence involved in learning a new motor skill. According to Fitts (1962), there are three phases involved: cognitive, fixative, and autonomous. In the first phase, the "teacher" provides information about the new behavior and models it. The "learner" then thinks about the information and the model and develops a plan for how he will perform the behavior. When he has completed his planning, he then attempts the behavior. This continues until the behavior is relatively stable. The second phase, fixative, consists of the "learner" practicing the new behavior until there are no errors. In the final phase, autonomous, the speed of production is increased to the point where it is functional as a part of a larger behavioral unit. This sequence reflects what occurs when we teach the client a new speech behavior:

1. We provide a model and information about the behavior.

2. The client then thinks about it and forms a plan for how to imitate the model.

3. The client then attempts to imitate the model as he perceived it.

When the model has been accurately imitated, we move into the next phase of therapy, where the behavior is practiced until it occurs consistently with no errors. The next step in therapy is to increase the speed of production of the new behavior so that it fits into the larger behavioral unit—the client's speech.

Cognitive Learning

There are many theories and concepts that could be classified as cognitive learning. In essence, these theories and concepts assume that the thinking or cognitive process of the individual is involved in such activities as perception, problem solving through insight, decision making, processing information, and comprehension. Of all the various aspects of cognition, the most important ones to the speech clinician are memory and problem solving.

There are two types of memory: long-term and short-term. Long-term memory concerns the retention of information for long periods of time. This type of information, such as your name and telephone number, is maintained since it is rehearsed often. For example, long-term memory of a person's age fades after he or she reaches age 39 because he is not asked to recall it as frequently. When information is not rehearsed or used, it is forgotten. Think back to your class in anatomy and see what information you remember. You will probably remember only the information you have recalled or used as a clinician. Or, consider a class where you crammed, not to learn the information but just to get a passing grade in the course; you probably do not remember any of the information or, perhaps, even the name of the course. This latter example leads us to short-term memory.

Short-term memory consists of bits of information that we retain only for a short period of time since it is not needed over an extended time period. We use our short-term memory to remember a telephone number we have looked up long enough to dial it. We also use it, or should use it, at parties where we are introduced to people and remember their names only for the duration of the party. This type of information is not vital to our survival, so we do not commit it to our long-term memory system.

Both forms of memory are important to therapy. If we teach a client a new behavior or concept, we expect him to remember it over an extended period of time. As a result, if the client does not have long-term memory, we have great difficulty with our therapy. Such clients come into therapy each time as though it were the first session because clinical progress is dependent on long-term memory.

Short-term memory has a more immediate impact on our therapy. We give our clients instructions such as "Put the spoon in the cup" and "Hand me the knife," or we ask them to repeat messages such as "Repeat after me, 'I found a fat frog.'" If a client cannot retain this information long enough to perform the task, therapy is going to be extremely difficult.

The other aspect of cognitive learning that has an impact on our therapy is problem solving through insight. When a person is confronted with a problem, something they do not understand, they compare it with their memories of similar experiences, information they have, and other cognitive resources. In other words, they think about the problem in terms of their own knowledge, memories, and experiences. If their thinking results in a solution to the problem, it does so very quickly. Suddenly, the solution is very clear, and all the factors involved are obvious. The best way to explain this is to let you experience it. Please look at the word games that follow. Each of the three games represents a term or phrase that a speech clinician would use. The solution to the game lies in the relationship between the words, the spacing of the words, or some other such factor. Do not take the words at face value. See if you can do some problem solving by insight.

1. PAL ATE

2. PITUPCH

3. ARTIK, ARTIK, ARTIK

I hope that you had some success in finding a solution to the word games. If not, you are going to have to look in Appendix C for the solutions. You will also find a few more word games there to practice on.

The gaining of insight is very important to our therapy. We confront our clients with many problems for which they must find solutions. We present them with a variety of stimuli that they must integrate and gain insight into before they can use the information. We present them with a model of a sound, give them some information about how it is made, and then expect them to be able to produce it. They must integrate all this information and achieve insight into the relationships before they can respond appropriately. We give clients numerous rules concerning phonology and expect this to influence their speech production. However, there will be no influence until the clients gain insight into the relationships among the rules we give them and their speech. This is a part of verbal comprehension: the complete understanding of what is presented on a verbal level. It involves understanding not only the individual words, but also their relationships and the concepts they convey. Perhaps we achieve comprehension and understanding only when the client gains insight into the problems we present to him.

Establishing a Clinical Vocabulary

As I mentioned earlier, one of the main problems we have when we discuss therapy is the lack of a vocabulary that communicates clinical concepts. We are currently limited to a vocabulary that describes only our clinical behaviors. Before we go further in the discussion of the clinical process, it is important that we establish a clinical vocabulary so we can communicate on a concept level.

The Cognitive–Behavioral Approach

The cognitive aspect of our cognitive–behavioral therapy is eclectic in nature in that it utilizes concepts from a number of learning paradigms. The cognitive–behavioral approach to therapy may appear to be unique because it combines cognitive learning with non–cognitive conditioning procedures. To some, this may seem to be a contradiction, but, in truth, the client's cognitions cannot be prevented or ignored. They are a part of any treatment procedure, regardless of the intent of the theoretic approach. Our approach is not unique; it is a reflection of the Cognitive Behavior Modification movement started by Meichenbaum (1977).

In getting a new behavior to occur, we use a number of techniques that depend on the client's cognitions. We may model the new behavior, but the client must be aware of it, perceive it, think about it, and then shift it from abstract perception to concrete production. We may physically guide the client's tongue in the production of a sound. Again, the client must be cognitively involved in applying this information when he attempts to make the correct production of the sound. In this context, the client is constantly involved in therapy on a cognitive level.

We must also look at cognition from the standpoint of the cognitive involvement of the clinician. If the clinician is performing her therapy in a reflexive, rote manner, she is probably not deeply involved on a cognitive level. Good therapy calls for the clinician to be totally involved on a cognitive level, evaluating the client's responses, determining an appropriate response to the client's behavior, and changing the clinical strategy if the client fails to respond or comprehend. And let us not forget that the clinician must be aware of the client's attitudes, emotions, feelings, and needs. These factors play an important part in therapy, and the clinician must take them into consideration not only in planning a treatment program but also as treatment progresses. In some instances, the treatment program might focus on the client's emotional issues. This clinical approach will be discussed in detail in Chapter 11. In any event, there must be a total commitment of the thinking process to the ongoing clinical interaction. Effective and efficient therapy is hard work on the part of the clinician as well as on the part of the client.

Special Semantic Problems

Any attempt to bridge the gap between theory and therapy results in the compromise of one or both positions. In our cognitive–behavioral approach, both are compromised. However, I have attempted to make the compromises as palatable as possible for both the theoretician and the practitioner. Attempts to simplify complex systems often lead to oversimplification. This is an inherent problem with our cognitive behavioral approach. I can only hope that as you and I gain more clinical experience and deeper insight into principles and concepts of learning, we will expand and fill in the clinical framework presented in this book.

There are several terms we will be using that need to be discussed before you read their definitions. The terms *reinforce* and *punish* often cause confusion and misunderstanding, particularly the term *punish*. In much of the literature concerning operant conditioning, the terms *reward* and *penalty* are used as synonyms for *reinforce* and *punish*. We will use these terms since they are much clearer in meaning to most people. This terminology can be extremely important in those clinical environments where we are communicating with people such as teachers, occupational therapists, physical therapists, physicians, or clinical aides, who may not have a clear understanding of the terms *reinforce* and *punish*. The term *penalize* seems to have less of a negative connotation than does the term *punish*. Depending on the agency where the clinical services are offered, this distinction can be very important.

Continuing along in this vein, when we use reward or penalty, we set up different cognitive sets, or mental attitudes, in our clients. When we apply a reward, the client has a positive attitude and behaves in such a way as to get more rewards. However, when we apply a penalty, the client's attitude has a negative orientation, and he changes his behavior in order to escape from or avoid the penalty. We need terms to describe the different attitudes the client might have in therapy. This is important since we will be discussing clinical strategies that will purposely create these different attitudes. However, there are currently no standard terms we can use here. If we turn to clinical terminology, we find that many clinicians use the term *motivation* to describe a client's attitude toward therapy. However, motivation can be interpreted as a client being motivated to achieve rewards or to avoid penalties.

Two other terms that are related to these client attitudes are *approach* and *avoidance*. The positive mental attitude is approach and the negative attitude is avoidance. The positive mental attitude leads to approach behavior to achieve more rewards, while the negative mental attitude leads to the avoidance of penalties.

We will combine the terms into *approach motivation* and *avoidance motivation* and use these terms to describe the two attitudinal states we are discussing. When a behavior is followed by a positive consequence (reward), the client develops approach motivation, which results in the behavior being performed more often. When a behavior is followed by a negative consequence (penalty), the client develops avoidance motivation, which results in the behavior being performed less often.

We are now ready to assemble our clinical vocabulary. Because the cognitive–behavioral approach is eclectic, terms from several different learning paradigms are used. Read the following definitions carefully since some definitions include examples related to our cognitive–behavioral approach. The definitions will be expanded in later chapters, and clinical examples will be provided to further clarify the terms and concepts they represent.

Clinical Vocabulary

Behavior. A behavior is anything a person does. Overt behaviors are actions or movements that can be observed. Covert behaviors are thoughts or feelings that cannot be observed but are still considered behaviors. There is a concept known as the *dead man rule*, which indicates that anything a living person can do that a dead man cannot do is a behavior. This should give us room to operate.

Behaviors have three characteristics which we will be concerned with: their frequency of occurrence, their strength or intensity when they occur, and their duration. We will be manipulating these characteristics as we move through the clinical process.

Stimulus (S). A stimulus is anything that attracts a person's attention. It may be something inside the person, such as a headache, or something in their external environment, such as objects in a room. We will not view a stimulus as an event that elicits a behavior, but rather as an event that prompts or cues a behavior. The behavior may be either overt or covert.

Response (R). A response is the reaction a person has to a stimulus—a behavior. Responses include thinking about the stimulus, looking at an object in a room, imitating a speech behavior presented by the clinician, rewarding a client for a correct performance, and other such behaviors.

Antecedent Event. An antecedent event is any event that precedes the response; that is, the stimulus that prompts or cues a response to occur.

Modeling. Modeling is the demonstration of a behavior. We show the clients what we want them to do. This could include such diverse behaviors as the production of the [r] sound, maintaining eye contact, opening the jaw further during speech, slowing down the rate of speech, or using the correct syntax. This is the demonstration of the behavior-change goal so that our clients know what we expect them to do.

Information. In our contact with the client, we can either provide for the client or request from the client two types of information. First, we can provide *behavioral* information that is concerned with the behavior we are attempting to teach. This type of information might include such things as telling the client to prolong the vowel when attempting to slow down the rate of speech or to hold the teeth closer together when attempting to make the [s] sound. We can also ask the client to repeat what we have said to make sure he understood us.

Second, we can provide *general* information. This might include a description of our therapy, therapy goals, and information designed to change attitudes or emotions. Again, we might ask the client to repeat what we have told him to determine his perception of what we said. We can also ask the client for information concerning his attitudes, emotions, and feelings regarding his communicative disorder. This is the basis of any counseling we might have to do with the client and is discussed in depth in Chapter 11, Counseling.

Guidance. Another term for guidance is *prompt*. There are four types of guidance that we use in therapy. We give *verbal* guidance in the form of hints or cues about the behavior. *Gestural* guidance involves gestures we make to prompt or cue a behavior to occur. We also use *environmental* guidance when we manipulate the environment so that it elicits the behavior, such as showing the client a picture. Finally, we use *physical* guidance, where we actually touch the client to assist in the performance of a behavior.

Contingent Event. A contingent event is any event that follows the response. This means either a pleasant event (reward) or an unpleasant event (penalty).

Reward (R +). *Reward* means the same thing as *reinforcement*. It is the positive event that occurs after a behavior is performed. If the event is truly rewarding to the client, the chances of the behavior occurring again are increased.

Penalty (P). *Penalty* means the same thing as *punishment*. It signifies the negative event that occurs after a behavior is performed. If the event is truly penalizing to the client, the chances of the behavior occurring again are decreased.

Extinguish. When reward for a behavior is withheld, the behavior will extinguish. That is, it will no longer occur, since the reward is no longer presented and the behavior no longer has a purpose. However, if the behavior has become self-rewarding, it will continue to occur since it is no longer dependent on an external reward.

Reward Schedule. When we use this term, we are referring to how often we re-ward a behavior. A *continuous* schedule means that we reward every occur-rence of a behavior. This provides fast learning, but the behavior is not very stable and will have a tendency to cease to occur when the reward is removed. With an *intermittent* schedule, we reward on a more random basis. There are two types of intermittent systems. In the *ratio* system, either fixed or variable, the reward is given based on the number of times the behavior has occurred. In the *interval* system, the determining factor for reward is time. Intermittent schedules are not as efficient for learning a behavior, but they make the behav-ior very stable, and the behavior will have a tendency to continue to occur even after the reward is removed.

Approach Motivation. Approach motivation represents a client's mental atti-tude that is focused on rewards. He will perform the behavior being rewarded more often in order to get more rewards.

Avoidance Motivation. This represents the mental attitude of the client that fo-cuses on penalties. He will perform the behavior being penalized less often in order to avoid the penalty.

Shaping. Shaping is the process of creating a new behavior in a client. As be-haviors more closely approximate the target behavior, they are rewarded, and through this process the new behavior is gradually shaped.

Significant Others (SOs). Significant others are people who are very important in the client's life. They may be the client's parents, spouse, close friend, or similar figure.

Token Economy. A token economy occurs when the client is initially rewarded with tokens, such as poker chips, which he can turn in at some later time for a more meaningful reward.

Stimulus Control. Stimuli can be manipulated in several ways. They can be gradually presented, gradually withdrawn, increased in number, or decreased in number, and their prompting role can be changed. This is *stimulus control*.

Fading. Fading is the gradual removal of a stimulus. Remember that when we reward a client, the reward is a stimulus to the client, and it can be gradually withdrawn (faded).

The Clinician–Client Interaction

The Transaction

The dynamics of the interaction between the clinician and the client can best be viewed as a continuous series of transactions. There are two basic types of these transactions: small talk and clinical. The small talk transaction is used to establish rapport or, in many instances, because the clinician forgot to plan therapy. Since the small talk transactions seem to come naturally to most clinicians, especially when they are not prepared for therapy, we will concern ourselves with the clinical transactions. These transactions can be illustrated by using some of the terms we have just defined and by showing them in proper sequential order. The first half of a transaction would appear like this:

▶ S–O–R

This represents the clinician presenting the stimulus (S) to the client (O = organism/cognition). The clinician might be modeling the correct production of the [k] sound. As the client hears and sees (perceives) the model, he will think about it (cognition) before he attempts to imitate it. When he does make his attempt to imitate it, we have his response (R). We now have completed one-half of the transaction. The clinician must now respond to the client, so we will expand the diagram.

▶ S–O–R/S–O–R

The first half of the diagram remains the same, but now we see that the response (R) of the client becomes the stimulus (S) for the clinician. As she hears and sees the client's response she must make some very important decisions and then respond to the client. This completes the first transaction of ongoing therapy, the first of a continuing series of transactions between the clinician and the client. To continue the interaction between the clinician and the client, we must again expand our diagram.

▶ (S–O–R/S–O–R)(S–O–R)

Now it is the clinician's turn to provide another (S) that will start the next transaction. When she evaluates the client's last response, she decides where the transaction should go and what she is going to say. Let us consider an example of this. In the first transaction, the client is attending and has responded with a sound that is a close approximation of the correct [k] sound. The clinician's response to the client's [k] production might be a reward such as "That was a good sound." She then starts the second transaction by saying, "Now, let's try it again. Listen—[k]." The (S) is then the repeating of the model of the [k] sound. The cycle starts over again with the client seeing and hearing the sound, thinking about it, and then trying it. This second response is another stimulus to which the clinician responds. We must expand the diagram one more step.

▶ (S–O–R/S–O–R)(S–O–R/S–O–R)

The clinician now makes her decision regarding the correctness of the sound and responds to the second attempt. We have two transactions completed. Perhaps it would be easier if we could visualize these clinical transactions in a circular form, such as seen in Figure 3.4.

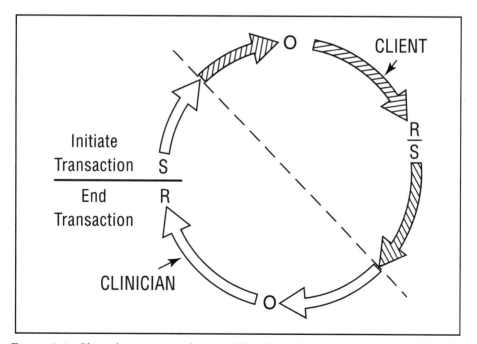

Figure 3.4. Clinical transaction diagram. The clinical transaction is initiated by the clinician's stimulus (S). The client thinks about the stimulus (O) and then responds (R). The client's response is the stimulus (S) for the clinician. She evaluates the client's stimulus (O) and then responds (R). This constitutes one clinical transaction. The clinician's next stimulus (S) initiates the next transaction.

Visualize these transactions as continuing around the circle, one time around for each succeeding transaction. Therapy, then, is like a string of beads, with each transaction building on and following the previous transaction. Each stimulus from the clinician is dependent on her evaluation of the client's performance in the previous transaction. If you carefully examine the previous example, you will recognize that the therapy transaction is a very complex interaction involving cognitive influence on the parts of both the client and the clinician. If the client is distracted from the transaction, therapy is no longer possible. This must be dealt with immediately so that therapy can proceed.

The client's lack of attention may be reflected in bodily posture, loss of eye contact, or general attitude. A need to go to the bathroom might be reflected in bodily positions or fidgeting. These signs are especially important to pick up on in order to prevent catastrophes (see Leith's Laws of Therapy in Appendix A). There are many factors that can influence the client's responses, and the clinician must be aware of them.

The cognitive involvement on the part of the clinician includes attending to all of her senses during the transactions. Feedback from the client takes many forms and occurs at any time in the transaction, not just during the client's response. The clinician must constantly monitor the client to pick up cues as to his level of attention, comprehension, and so forth.

During the clinical interactions, the clinician will also have to determine what role she will play. If she is a flexible and adaptable clinician, she will have several clinical roles, each depending on the actions and needs of the client. Being cognitively involved in the interactions, she is aware of the different roles the client plays from day to day or even from transaction to transaction. She must adapt to the client's role to maintain control over the therapy. For example, if a child is unruly and challenging the clinician, she might have to assume the authority role. If the client is upset and hurt, the clinician might assume the comforting role. If an adult client becomes too friendly, stepping over the professional line, the clinician might have to assume the professional role. If a client is not performing up to his capabilities, the clinician might well adopt a demanding role.

There are many clinical "hats" that we wear. We are one person to one client and another person to another client. Our role is dependent on the relationship we have with the client and the client's needs at a particular time. We should be aware of the various clinical roles we play, recognizing each for its value so that we can quickly apply the appropriate role.

Clinical Testing

One of the most important factors to consider is that the transactions between the clinician and the client are TEST situations. The clinician is continually testing (a) the client's response in terms of its correctness, (b) the effects of rewards and penalties on the frequency of occurrence of behaviors, and (c) the client's levels of approach motivation and avoidance motivation. This testing is vital since it, and it alone, determines whether a transaction must be repeated or whether the therapy can move ahead into the next phase of learning.

The client's responses give the clinician insight into the cognitions of the client and tells her if she can continue working on the speech behavior or if she must shift the clinical focus to the client's attending behavior. The responses help the clinician detect whether any problems are occurring in therapy. Problem solving cannot take place until the clinician is aware of and carefully defines any problems.

During the transaction, the clinician must determine how she will respond to the client. It is imperative that there be a response from the clinician, some sort of acknowledgment that at least indicates that the clinician was aware the client responded. One way to extinguish a newly created behavior in therapy is not to respond to it. If there is no consequence for a behavior, there is no reason to perform the behavior. For example, students have approach motivation and study for examinations because there is a consequence—the reward of a good grade. Or could it be avoidance motivation—to avoid a failing grade? If there is no consequence for a speech behavior, no response from the clinician, the client will have no approach motivation to achieve a reward or avoidance motivation to avoid a penalty.

Later in the clinical process we will withdraw the reward, but this will be for a special reason that we will discuss in another chapter. For now, we view the clinician's response to the client's behavior as a vital component in the clinical interaction between the clinician and the client. It is an essential part of the learning process, especially when the new behavior is just being introduced.

The Clinical Interaction Model

The Clinical Interaction Model (CIM) is a clinical communications model and was developed by combining various aspects of the learning theories with the clinician–client transaction (S–O–R/S–O–R; see Figure 3.5). In each transaction the clinician has three clinical tasks she must perform if the transaction is to be completed. She must provide the initial stimulus, evaluate the client's response, and deliver her response. We will discuss each of these tasks.

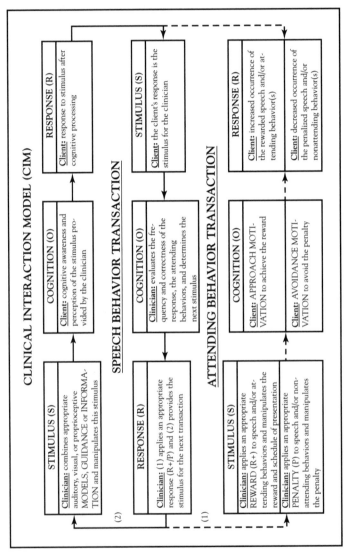

Figure 3.5. Clinical Interaction Model (CIM). Clinical Interaction Model (CIM) illustrates the two clinical transactions that are occurring simultaneously in therapy. The clinician is attending to the speech behaviors of the client as well as to his attending behaviors. The focal point of therapy is the speech behavior, but if the attending behavior becomes a problem, the clinician can focus her therapy on the client's motivation and attending behaviors. Her response to the client, either reward or penalty, is very critical. It not only affects the occurrences of the client's speech behaviors but also influences the client's motivation in therapy.

Antecedent Events: The Clinician's Stimulus

Modeling. One of the ways we can make therapy more efficient is to present the client with the behavior change goal. We can show or model the behavior, demonstrating or modeling articulation sounds, forms of syntax, new voice quality, fluency controls for the stutterer, and so forth. Modeling is one of our most important teaching techniques and has been used by speech clinicians for many years. Remember, this is also the way many speech clinicians learn the *how* of therapy, by observing the models provided by their instructors.

Guidance. As pointed out earlier, guidance is leading or directing the client to the correct behavior. The guidance could be verbal, gestural, environmental, or physical. We provide verbal guidance when we say to a client, "Can you make the sound just like I did?" or "How do we ask for water?" These are prompts to get the client to produce a behavior without modeling it. Gestural guidance would include those facial expressions and body or hand gestures we use to prompt a behavior (e.g., if a client has a vocal pitch problem and we use a hand gesture to cue the client to raise or lower his pitch, we are using gestural guidance). Environmental guidance occurs when we manipulate the stimuli in the client's surroundings in such a way that the desired behavior occurs. For example, if we are working on sucking behavior, we might prompt it by having a glass of juice with a straw in it sitting on a table in front of the client. This is also referred to as indirect therapy, since the clinician is working through the environment to prompt the behavior to occur. An example of physical guidance is the manipulation of the client's mouth as in the moto-kinesthetic method of articulation therapy.

Information. We can provide our clients with two types of information: *behavioral* and *general*. Behavioral information is used to supplement the model of the behavior. We can give the client instructions on how he should hold his mouth or on tongue placement. This type of information is directly related to the performance of the behavior we are teaching. General information can occur at any time during therapy. It is any information that the clinician gives the client that is not directly related to speech behavior. This includes setting up future appointments, giving instructions on home programs, and so forth.

Evaluation: The Clinician's Cognitions

The clinician has four important decisions to make before she can respond to the client. First, she must evaluate the correctness of the response. This will determine whether she will reward the production or penalize it. Second, she must determine whether the correct response is occurring more often and the incorrect response is occurring less often. This will tell her whether her rewards and penalties are functioning as they should or if she needs to change them. Third, she needs to evaluate the attentiveness of the client to therapy. If the client is not attending, then she must reevaluate her reward and her penalty since these are her tools to create approach motivation and avoidance motivation in the client. Fourth, she must determine how she will respond at the end of this transaction and initiate the next one. These decisions are dependent on what she has found in her testing. She may move ahead with therapy if the client's response is satisfactory. She may have to repeat the last transaction if the response is unsatisfactory.

If there are problems in therapy, they will be discovered by the clinician's evaluation. Clinical problems usually center around the correctness of responses, the frequency of occurrence of responses, and the client's attention to therapy. These problems are directly related to the appropriateness of the clinician's stimulus and response. If the stimulus is not appropriate, it will result in incorrect behavioral responses by the client. If the reward response is not appropriate, it will not create approach motivation and the results will be no increase in the frequency of occurrence of the appropriate behavior and a lack of interest and motivation in therapy.

The answers to these problems involve modifying either the stimulus or the reward response. If the problem is consistently incorrect responses by the client, the stimulus may be too complex for the client or inappropriate in some other way. The stimulus can be modified by the amount, duration, and complexity of information, guidance, and modeling. It can also be reviewed to see whether the objectives being taught can be addressed in another way. In any event, the stimulus should be modified and then tested again in the next transaction.

Another factor that could create problems is moving too fast in therapy. This results from improper assessment of the correctness of the behavior. Care should be taken to make sure that the behavioral performance is closely evaluated in each transaction.

If the fault is with the reward, the reward should be changed. Perhaps the client is satiated with the reward. The client must be interested in getting the reward, or it has no value as a motivator. When the client is again interested in the reward, the frequency of behavioral performance will increase, and he will attend to therapy, since he is motivated to get the reward.

In addition to making the four decisions and resolving any problems related to them, the clinician must also be aware of the client's attitudes, emotions, and feelings during the transactions. As long as these factors are not negatively influencing the treatment program, the clinician does no more than monitor them. But if any of these factors begin to interfere with therapy, the clinician will have to deal with them. In fact, the basic therapy plan may have to be temporarily set aside while the clinician deals with, for example, the client's attitude.

We need to recognize that negative attitudes, emotions, and feelings contribute to problematic behavior in the therapy room. When behaviors occur that disrupt the therapy interactions, the clinician must regain control. The question arises, "Who is in charge of the therapy program?" The clinician must be in charge, or no learning will take place. In order to regain control, the clinician must deal directly with the interfering behaviors. This is accomplished through the use of an appropriate clinical role (e.g., an authoritarian role), facial expressions showing strong disapproval, stern requests that the behavior in question be stopped, or even some form of penalty for the performance of the behavior. The clinician cannot be vague with her demands or her threats. The client must know that she means business and that it would be wise to stop performing the behavior. In some instances, this is a test of wills between the client and clinician. There are those clients who need to see how far they can push the clinician; if the clinician gives in to the pressure, all control is lost.

When the clinician is working in a group therapy environment with younger children, all the control advice given above is tripled. The children can play off one another, reinforcing the interfering behaviors; in such situations, the clinician quickly discovers what mob rule is.

Another cognitive evaluation the clinician should make involves the client's attitude toward her. Many clinicians do not understand the difference between the terms *like* and *respect*. They feel the client must like them, so they yield to the client's demands. When this happens, they lose control of the interaction, and the client loses some respect for them. In my own clinical experience, I have felt the most important part of my relationship with a client was for the client to respect me. If I could achieve respect and have the client like me too, all the better. But I could not accept the client liking me while not respecting me. If you are a bit confused with all this, let me ask you to think of a person you know and like, who is pleasant to be around, but whom you really do not respect as a person. Now, think of another person you have a lot of respect for but do not necessarily like being around. And, finally, think of someone you both like and respect. Clearly, there are significant differences.

Control over therapy interactions is easiest if the client both likes and respects you. You can still maintain control if the client just respects you but does not particularly like you. However, if the client likes you but has no respect for you, you will have difficulty in gaining and maintaining control over clinical interactions.

Before we move on from the topic of the clinician's cognitions and controlling problematic behavior, let us consider another source of negative behavior in the therapy room—you. Negative attitudes, emotions, and feelings toward the client, the therapeutic interaction, your supervisor, or other persons involved in your clinical activities could bring about problematic behaviors on your part. You must monitor your own behaviors in the clinical environment and make certain they do not interfere with the effectiveness and efficiency of your clinical activities. If you are not able to extract your personal problems from your clinical activities, your therapy will be ineffective and so will your interactions with others involved.

Finally, we need to recognize that it is our cognitive evaluation of the client's behavioral performances that determines our response to the performance. This is an extremely important aspect of therapy. Our evaluations must be done carefully and thoroughly if they are to accurately reflect the behavioral performance. We do not want to reward incorrect behaviors or penalize correct behaviors. If, based on our evaluation, we use a reward, we create approach motivation in the client. He is motivated to get the reward and will attend to therapy and perform the appropriate speech behavior so he can get the reward. On the other hand, if our evaluation is negative and we use a penalty, we create avoidance motivation in the client. He is motivated to avoid the penalty, and will attend to therapy and not perform the incorrect speech behavior that results in the penalty. Motivation, in one form or another, is essential for successful therapy.

These contingent events are powerful incentives, and they are under our control. Careful planning and observation on our part will make rewards and penalties very effective teaching tools.

Contingent Events: The Clinician's Response

Before discussing the clinician's response, I would like to discuss a little deeper the principles and concepts involved here. In any clinical transaction, when we use rewards we are encouraging a behavior to occur more frequently and when we use penalties we are discouraging the performance of a behavior. Some clinicians use only rewards to establish and habituate the new speech behavior. This is inefficient, since therapy is then completely dependent on the habit strength of the new behavior in replacing the incorrect behavior. Not only does the old behavior have great habit strength built up over years of performance, it also gains habit strength each time it is performed, even in error. The new behavior must compete with the old behavior for performance, and the old behavior is stronger and more automatic. When the new behavior is finally established, it may be more the result of maturity than therapy.

Cognitive–behavioral therapy also focuses on rewards, but only in the early stages of therapy. Once the correct behavior is learned and begins to occur automatically, we introduce penalty into the therapy interaction. We reward the occurrences of the new behavior and penalize the occurrences of the incorrect behavior. By doing this we are not only actively encouraging the new behavior to occur but also actively discouraging the occurrence of the incorrect behavior. For example, the client is given a token for each occurrence of the new behavior but a token is taken back when the incorrect behavior is performed. The client has approach motivation to get the tokens and avoidance motivation to keep from losing tokens. This results in the new behavior's frequency of occurrence increasing and the incorrect behavior's frequency of occurrence decreasing.

It is very important to remember that this form of reward/penalty interactive therapy is not introduced until the client can perform the new behavior. This form of therapy is most effective in encouraging the habituation and generalization of the new behavior. Consider the following clinical example. The client's original problem was a nasal voice. He was taught to produce a normal voice and this was rewarded to increase the frequency with which it occurred. Penalty was then introduced and the client was penalized each time he produced the nasal voice. The result of this was a reduction in the occurrence of the nasal voice. Each time he produced the good voice he received two types of rewards. The first reward was an R+, a positive reward for producing good voice quality. The second reward came from the fact that by producing the good voice he avoided the penalty. This was an R−, a negative reward for the good voice quality.

Both approach and avoidance motivation are now operating, resulting in dramatic increases in the frequency of the correct voice quality. This is partially the result of the client not producing the nasal quality in order to avoid the penalty. This is the carrot and stick principle, encouraging forward progress both by dangling a carrot in front and discouraging stopping by applying a stick to the other end. Your therapy has the same principles operating: rewards to encourage one behavior (normal voice) and penalties to discourage another (nasal voice).

Reward. As mentioned earlier, reward is the same thing as reinforcement. It is an event that occurs after the behavior is performed, and the client views it as a positive event. If the client feels that the contingent event is a reward, the probability that the behavior will occur again is increased. The client is highly motivated to get the reward and will perform the appropriate behavior to be rewarded. Approach motivation is important in therapy. There is a danger here, though. Many times, clinicians decide that something is rewarding to the client when it actually is not. We cannot determine if something is rewarding until we see the effect it has on the client's behavior. If we respond to a client in a certain way several times and the behavior we are responding to increases in frequency of occurrence, then, and only then, can we say that the response is rewarding. Remember, the reward is for the client, not you. You may like chocolate and enjoy eating it; however, if your client has an allergic reaction and breaks out in a rash, the chocolate is not a reward to him. His only rewarding behavior is scratching. Obviously, we must predetermine what we are going to use as a reward, and we base this decision on our past clinical experience. We must also remember to observe the effect of our reward on the client to see if our decision was correct.

The importance of observing the effect of the reward on the behavior is clearly illustrated in a published report by a clinician (Van Riper, 1957). In this report, the clinician indicated that he rewarded stuttering behavior by having a female clinician kiss the stutterer each time he had a block. The occurrence of stuttering behavior all but disappeared, and the clinician then concluded that stuttering behavior does not follow the operant principle of increase in frequency of occurrence with contingent reward. The clinician was observant and noted that the behavior changed in frequency of occurrence. But he failed to realize that the kiss from the female clinician was functioning as a penalty rather than as a reward. The clinician based his determination of a reward on his own values, but his "guess" was wrong. Even though "kiss therapy" appears to reduce stuttering, I would hesitate to recommend it. The treatment program might create a few problems for both you and your client.

There are two types of rewards we can give our clients: Primary rewards meet basic needs such as food and water; secondary rewards have more of a social impact and are learned, such as telling the child "good" after a production or patting him on the head. We must be concerned with both the strength of the reward and how appropriate it is for our clinical setting. If someone offered you 50¢ to type a 10-page paper for him, you would probably turn down the offer. But if he offered $500, you would rush to your typewriter. This is approach motivation! The strength of the reward is very important and is determined by the client. If there is good rapport between the client and the clinician, the reward is strengthened, since the clinician is an important person to the client. Furthermore, it is important to remember that what may be a powerful reward for you may not be so powerful for your client. The appropriateness of the reward is also very important. If the reward is a very chewy gum candy, therapy must wait until it is eaten, which might take a considerable amount of time. If we do use a consumable reward, we must decide when it is to be consumed— during or after therapy.

We also must consider the timing of the reward. If there is a lengthy period of time between the performance of the behavior and the presentation of the reward, the association between the reward and the behavior may be lost. The client might have performed another behavior in the meantime, and, although the reward is contingent upon the earlier behavior, the more recent behavior is the one that is rewarded. For example, the client performs the appropriate speech behavior and follows this by scratching his nose. The clinician then gives the client the reward. The clinician is now rewarding the scratching, which increases in frequency of occurrence. *To be effective, rewards must be given immediately after the desired behavior has been performed.*

Finally, we need to consider the reward's schedule of presentation. If we reward each and every performance of the behavior, this is a *constant reward schedule*. The ratio here is 1:1; for every response there is a reward. This leads to rapid learning, but when the reward is removed, there is also rapid extinction. The behavior disappears quickly without the reward. An alternative is the *intermittent reward schedule*. If we reward every third performance of the behavior, we are using a fixed ratio; that is, a ratio of 3:1. The fixed ratio can be varied according to the client's response.

It is very important to recognize that when we move from a 1:1 ratio (continuous reward) to a 2:1 ratio (intermittent reward), we are actually going from a 100% reward schedule to a 50% reward schedule. This is quite a large step— too large for some clients. This difference can be reduced if we adjust the ratio by adding zeros (e.g., changing the 1:1 ratio to a 10:10 ratio). This is actually the same ratio, but now we can manipulate it into smaller steps by moving to a 10:9 ratio. We are now rewarding 9 of 10 performances, or a 90% schedule of reward. We can then adjust it downward to a 10:8 ratio, a 10:7 ratio, and so forth. These smaller steps of reward withdrawal may be necessary for some clients.

We can also use a variable ratio. This means that we might reward the third, fifth, and ninth performances. There is no set number of performances that must occur between rewards. You might even reward several performances in a row and then skip one. Intermittent reward is not as efficient in terms of learning a behavior quickly, but it does make the behavior extremely stable in terms of continued existence after the reward is removed. Behaviors learned under this schedule of reward are almost impossible to extinguish. Both continuous and intermittent schedules are important in the clinical process, as we shall see in later chapters.

The *fixed interval* and *variable interval* schedules have limited use for the speech clinician. However, we can use these techniques to work on the duration of a behavior. For example, we might use either the fixed or variable interval schedule to extend the time a child remains in his chair. The rewards extend the amount of time the child remains seated. We control this by varying the amount of time between rewards.

We cannot leave the concept of reward without acknowledging that there are many people who object to this form of therapy. Their objection is based upon the notion of bribing clients to work on their speech. The word "bribe" certainly does have negative connotations. I prefer to view the reward as payment for work. When I am confronted with the bribe concept, I ask the person if they are bribed where they work. The answer is always a firm "No." I then ask them if they would continue to work if their company or agency decided not to pay them. Again, the answer is "No." Now I ask you, the reader, is the salary a person receives for work a reward or a bribe? When we reward a client for work, it is not a bribe; it is a reward that the client has earned through his effort. Then again, who really cares what the motive is for the client as long as he is learning to perform the desired behavior?

Penalty. When a behavior is penalized it tends to occur less often. We focus our therapy on the production of the correct behavior, and we often tend to ignore productions of the incorrect behavior. Extinction theory indicates that if a behavior has no contingent event, it will no longer occur. However, there are pitfalls here, and extinction is a slow and rather impractical process for the speech clinician.

Many clinicians respond to incorrect productions by telling the client, "That was not very good, let's try it again." The clinician is providing feedback to the client that the production was incorrect. This is a form of penalty and will result in the decrease in the frequency of occurrence of the incorrect behavior. The client will have avoidance motivation to avoid the penalty and will not perform the behavior that results in the penalty. This is much more efficient than waiting for the incorrect response to extinguish over time.

We must take the same precautions using penalty that we took using reward. We must determine if our response is truly a penalty, control the strength of the penalty, and be concerned with the appropriateness of the penalty. To determine if the response is a penalty, we must determine its effect on the behavior. We also must be careful not to apply too great of a penalty. This can create problems with morale. And, of course, we must be careful not to use a penalty that is not appropriate to our clinical setting. Last, but not least, we must be consistent in applying the penalty.

There are two basic forms of penalty. We can administer a penalty, such as making the client pick up things he has thrown on the floor or making him stop and repeat a sound if he has made it incorrectly. We can also penalize a client by taking something positive away from him, such as removing a token when he makes the sound incorrectly. If the client has earned 20 tokens to purchase a reward after therapy and we take one away, this is a penalty. Knowing that if he makes the incorrect production he will lose one token, the client will have avoidance motivation and will want to avoid the penalty by not making the incorrect production. To make this more meaningful, consider what your response would be if every time you were late for class or late for work, you lost five of our society's tokens ($5, since our monetary system is a token economy). I doubt if you would be late again. You would have avoidance motivation to escape this penalty.

As with rewarding our clients, there are also many people who object to the concept of penalizing a client. In fact, there is a more negative reaction to penalty as a teaching tool than there is to reward. You can always be kind to another person, but it is difficult to be unkind. People often confuse being unkind with administering a penalty. I find it very interesting that all parents use some form of penalty as they raise their children, but they then object to the use of penalty in other learning environments.

Sometimes we can be very unkind by not penalizing a child. We are not providing the child with a learning experience. When we stop to think about it, much of our own learning was based on the avoidance of penalty. When I learned to ride a bicycle, one of the strongest factors in learning to balance the bike was to avoid the cuts and bruises that were a part of falling. And who cannot remember spankings? Penalty is a very important part of human learning. Clearly, however, the form of penalty we are using in therapy is not physical in nature.

Extinction. We cannot conclude the discussion on the clinician's response without considering extinction. Extinction of a behavior occurs when there is no longer a contingent event (a reward) and the behavior ceases to exist because it has no purpose. According to operant principles, this is the only way a behavior can be extinguished because penalty only reduces the occurrence of the behavior to an extremely low level. However, it is important to recognize that many operant principles, such as extinction, are mainly theoretical and effective only when applied to animals within the carefully controlled environment of the laboratory. This is not to say that the principles cannot be applied to humans; however, we must recognize that there are many differences between animals in laboratories and our clients in social environments. Cognitions and cognitively based values are variables that often interfere with principles such as extinction. We must use these principles with caution and carefully observe the results of our actions to determine the effect we have had. An example will make the extinction principle more realistic.

A father gives his son a small handsaw for his fourth birthday. The father's hobby is woodworking, and he wants to get his son involved in it. The next day the child takes the saw and begins to saw one of the legs off the grand piano. The mother, who has had a course in behavioral psychology, is observing the scene. She remembers that if there is no reward, the behavior will extinguish. So she ignores the behavior. The child continues to saw on the piano leg, and eventually two things are indeed extinguished: the piano when it falls and the child when the piano falls on him. What went wrong? The mother failed to realize that the behavior itself was rewarding to the child. Her response was not part of the paradigm.

Withholding rewards and other attempts at extinguishing behaviors will be marginally successful at best. If you attempt to use this principle in your therapy you should understand its limitations. Perhaps you should attempt to substitute a more adaptive behavior for the nonadaptive behavior, rather than merely attempting to extinguish it. This is the approach used in this book.

The CIM and the Clinical Process

The CIM is a clinical communication model and applies to all interactions with the client, significant others, and other professionals. However, its main focus is on the interactions in the actual treatment phases of the clinical process (i.e., getting the new behavior to occur, habituating the new behavior, and generalizing the new behavior). To give you an overview of how the CIM relates to each of these phases of therapy, all factors were combined and are shown in Figure 3.6. The evaluation and planning phase of therapy is not included in the figure because of the unique role of the CIM in that phase. That will be covered in Chapter 6, which deals with the evaluation and planning aspect of the clinical process.

"CIM AND THE CLINICAL PROCESS"

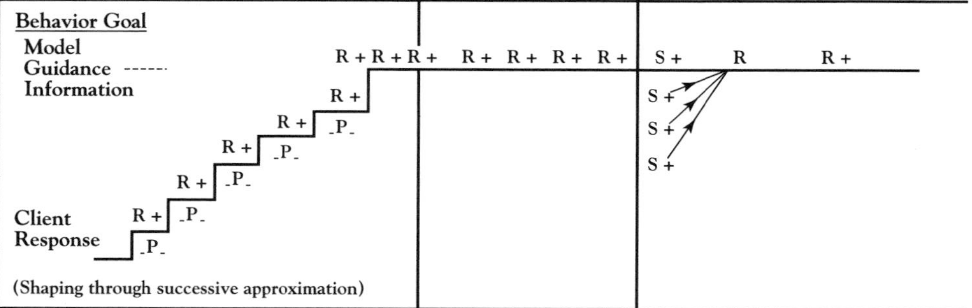

	Getting the New Behavior to Occur	Habituating the New Behavior	Generalizing the New Behavior (other environments)
	Behavior Goal Model Guidance ----- Information R + _P_ R + _P_ R + _P_ R + _P_ Client R + _P_ Response (Shaping through successive approximation)	R + R + R + R + R + R + R + R + R + Withdrawal of R + to test habituation	S + R R + s + s + s + Generalizing the response to other stimuli (other contexts, environments). S + cue for correct behavior. Withdraw R + to test habituation. (Applied by significant others if available)
BEHAVIORAL TECHNIQUES AND SYSTEMS	1. Modeling 2. Guidance 3. Information 4. Stimulus Manipulation 5. Reward 6. Penalty 7. Shaping 8. Token Economy	Withdrawal of R + to test habituation	Generalizing the response to other stimuli (other contexts, environments). S + cue for correct behavior. Withdraw R + to test habituation. (Applied by significant others if available)
REWARD SCHEDULE	Constant R + through Shaping	Initial intermittent R + and then withdrawal of R + to test habituation	Initial constant R +, shift to intermittent R +, then withdrawl of R + to test habituation. (Applied by significant others if available)

Figure 3.6. CIM and the clinical process. Although the CIM applies in each step of the clinical process, different techniques and procedures are emphasized in each step. This figure presents an overview of the clinical process and shows which techniques and procedures are emphasized in each step.

Figure 3.6 is a map of where we are going in future chapters as we deal with therapy. It will take on added significance as we progress with our discussion and will eventually serve as a handy reference that will provide you with an overview of your own therapy. As you examine the figure, note that the clinical techniques and procedures used by the clinician are listed under each step. For example, under the step "Getting the New Behavior to Occur," eight techniques and procedures are listed. These are the techniques and procedures that we will use in our CIM for this step in the clinical process.

CHAPTER

4

MANIPULATION AND MOTIVATION: THE M & M FACTORS

◆ Synopsis

One of the most important functions of the Clinical Interaction Model (CIM) is to provide the clinician with a means of establishing and maintaining client motivation and attention. This is achieved through the clinician's ability to manipulate her stimulus and response in the CIM. Without motivation, there is no attention, and without attention, there is no learning.

More general stimuli, such as the clinician herself or other things in the client's environment, can be conditioned so that they prompt or cue behaviors to occur or not to occur. These stimuli are manipulated to get behaviors to generalize outside the therapy environment and to eliminate unwanted behaviors that might interfere with therapy.

The flexibility and adaptability of the CIM is nowhere more apparent than when considering the many possible variations of the clinician's stimuli and responses. It is this ability to manipulate the stimulus and the response that makes it possible to tailor the CIM to each client's individual needs and to every clinical situation. The CIM allows the clinician to manipulate both the stimulus and the response within each transaction and, thus, provides her with a means of constantly monitoring and controlling the client's motivation. Motivation is the source of attention; together, motivation and attention form the foundation of learning. Without them, learning cannot take place.

In a more general way, we also need to consider the stimulus as any thing or event in the client's environment that attracts his attention (see the definition of stimulus in Chapter 3). The clinician, as well as other stimuli in the client's environment, can be conditioned and given special roles to prompt or cue behaviors to either occur or not to occur. These conditioned stimuli are important tools in the generalization of new speech behaviors or the elimination of old speech behaviors. The manipulation of stimulus roles to influence the occurrence of behaviors is called *stimulus control* and is an extremely important part of therapy.

Stimulus Manipulation with the CIM

Stimulus Control

Antecedent events can be manipulated and used clinically in special ways called stimulus control, which is important in all phases of the clinical process, especially generalizing the new behavior. The client becomes conditioned to the various stimuli in his environment and *these conditioned stimuli* then play a very important and unique role in the client's learning experience.

Stimulus Roles

We have discussed a stimulus as anything in the environment that attracts the attention of the client and brings about a reaction. There are an unlimited number of stimuli in the client's environment, but for the sake of our discussion, we will limit ourselves to three general types of stimuli. The first general type of stimuli are the people in the client's environment—all the people who interact with the client. We will also consider here what these people do, such as their verbal statements, their gestures and expressions, and so forth. The people are the source of many sub-stimuli. The second general type of stimuli are speaking situations the client experiences. These are special speaking situations that, particularly for the client who stutters, elicit an emotional response. Speaking situations include both specific speaking experiences, such as speaking before groups, and general ones, such as at home or school. The third general type of stimuli are objects in the client's environment, such as the tape recorder in the clinic room, or, for the stutterer, the telephone. We will now extend the concept of these stimuli to include the special roles that they assume after they have been associated with a specific contingent event.

Conditioned Stimuli

When a stimulus is consistently associated with a reward or a penalty the stimulus becomes conditioned. That is, the stimulus takes on a special characteristic or role, cuing the client as to what the outcome will be if a particular behavior is performed. These stimuli are known as *discriminative stimuli,* and they do not elicit a response like a tap on the knee elicits a knee jerk. Rather, they provide the client with a clue as to what is going to happen if he performs the behavior associated with the stimulus. These cues have a definite influence on the probability of the behavior occurring. Let us consider some general examples of discriminative stimuli.

Positive stimuli. There are those stimuli that have been conditioned to a positive outcome—a reward. We will refer to these conditioned stimuli as *positive stimuli* or S+. A steak on a platter has become an S+ to most of us, signifying that if we sit down and eat the steak, the outcome will be rewarding. This stimulus was not always a conditioned stimulus. It only assumed the role of an S+ after we had eaten and enjoyed the first steak and made the association between the steak and the reward of eating it. (We will ignore the penalty of paying for the steak since this ruins the analogy.) We also learned in this manner to answer the telephone. The telephone ring means nothing to the very young child. But when the telephone ringing is associated with answering the telephone and talking to someone we know, the reward changes the meaning of the telephone ringing.

Stimuli in the therapy environment quickly assume the role of S+ when rewards are presented. The clinician presents rewards for specific behaviors and when the client sees the clinician, her presence cues him such that, if he performs the behavior, he will be rewarded. Even the clinic room becomes associated with the reward and provides a cue for the correct behavior. This might tend to explain why most clinicians have experienced a client speaking extremely well in the therapy room and then reverting back to the old speech patterns as soon as he leaves the clinical environment. We are making great progress in the therapy room but the parents report that he is making no progress at home. When there is no S+ in his environment, there is no prompting for the correct speech behavior to occur.

Negative Stimuli. Other stimuli become associated with a negative outcome—a penalty. We will refer to these conditioned stimuli as *negative stimuli* or S−. An example of this is our first experience with a "No Left Turn" sign, where we received a traffic ticket. Either we had seen the sign and ignored it, or we had seen it but did not "register" its meaning. In any event, even though we plead our innocence with the traffic officer—telling him that the sign was positioned in such a way that it could not be seen from where our car was located, insisting that the sign was covered with snow even though it was July, and other equally valid arguments—we received a traffic ticket. This cost us between $40 and $60. After paying the fine, the sign took on significant meaning. We looked for "No Turn" signs and, indeed, did not turn. The sign cued us such that if we did turn we would get a ticket and have to pay another fine. We avoided the penalty of the fine by not performing the turn. We substituted another behavior—going straight ahead—and this allowed us to escape the penalty. There are innumerable examples of this type of learning in our lives, where we avoid penalties by performing different behaviors.

Just as with the S+, the clinician quickly assumes the S− role in the clinic room. If the client knocks all the materials off the clinic table onto the floor and the clinician then makes him pick up all the materials, she is applying the penalty and becomes associated with it. When the client enters the room, he is cued that if he knocks the materials off the clinic table, he will be penalized. Therefore, he performs another behavior to avoid the penalty; he does not knock the things off the clinic table. This same avoidance behavior occurs when the clinician assigns some sort of penalty to the production of the incorrect speech behavior. She becomes an S− for the incorrect production, cuing that if it is produced it will be penalized. The client then attempts to avoid the penalty by performing some other behavior. If the clinician has already taught the correct behavior, this would be the client's choice, since the correct behavior not only avoids the penalty but also achieves the reward.

Neutral Stimuli. So far, the clinician plays two stimulus roles in the clinic room: S+, prompting the correct production of the speech behavior, and S−, prompting the avoidance of the penalty by not producing the incorrect behavior. However, there is a third role that the stimulus can assume. This is the neutral stimuli or S0. This stimulus signals the client that there will be no reward for his behavior. Since the behavior is not rewarded, there is no reason for the behavior to exist. Thus, it extinguishes; it no longer occurs since it serves no function. The contingent event in this instance is zero (0).

Stimulus Manipulation

All stimuli can be manipulated by the clinician and can take several forms, such as changing the strength of the stimulus or shifting the role of the stimulus. Stimulus manipulation is a vitally important clinical procedure that we will use with the CIM in all phases of the clinical process. We will discuss each of the techniques involved in stimulus manipulation.

Shifting the Role of the Stimuli. Although a stimulus may have assumed the role of an S+, S−, or S0, these roles can be changed. If, for example, the parents have consistently penalized the client for his speech, their role is an S−. But if, because of counseling, they no longer react to the client's speech, their role will shift to S0. If on the other hand, the parents are rewarding the client's speech problem and maintaining it in the home environment, their role as S+ can be changed to that of S0 by removing the reward. The role of the stimulus can, therefore, be changed by associating the stimulus with a different contingent event. This ability to change becomes very important as we attempt to generalize the new speech behaviors into other environments. We can utilize the stimulus roles of the S0s in these environments to cue the new speech behaviors to occur in their presence. This is the key to carryover. The following illustration indicates that this role-shift is accomplished by associating the stimulus with a new contingent event. If the parents are only associated with penalty for a behavior, their role is S−. But if the parents are then associated with reward for the behavior, their role shifts to S+.

To Shift	Change Contingent Event
From/To	From/To
S−,S0/S+	P,0/R+
S+,S0/S−	R+/R+,0/P
S+,S−/S0	R+,P/0

Gradual Introduction of Stimuli. As we generalize a new behavior into other speaking environments, we may find that a certain stimuli is an S− and too threatening for the client. We will then have to gradually present the stimulus as the client adjusts to it. For example, a client who stutters might have great fear associated with speaking in front of groups (S−). For this client, we would gradually introduce such a speaking situation. We do this by starting with one listener where the client can perform satisfactorily (S+). We then add another listener. When the client has adjusted to this situation, we add another listener. This process is repeated so that we are gradually introducing the stimuli while keeping the talking situation at a level where the client can deal with it. We can gradually increase the frequency of the stimuli, the strength or intensity of the stimuli, or the duration of the stimuli. This procedure is as follows:

▶ s+ −R−R +
   S+ −R−R +
   S+ −R−R +
   S+ −R−R +

Gradual Withdrawal of Stimuli. This is also known as fading. We gradually with-draw the stimulus by presenting it less often, in a less complete form, or for a shorter period of time. We fade the speech model as the new speech behavior is learned. This helps make the behavior independent of the model. We can manipulate the frequency, intensity, or duration of the stimuli. This form of manipulation is seen below:

▶ S+ −R−R +
   S+ −R−R +
   S+ −R−R +
   s+ −R−R +
      −R−R +

Increase the Number of Stimuli. The clinician might also have to increase the number of stimuli in the client's environment. These stimuli (S+) would cue the new speech behavior to occur in other environments. The clinician must create more S+ in the client's nonclinical environment so that the new speech behaviors are cued to occur at home, at school, and on the job. This manipulation system is illustrated as follows:

▶ S+ = Clinical environment⎯⎯⎯R⎯⎯⎯R+
   S+ = Home environment
   S+ = School environment

Decrease the Number of Stimuli. The clinician can exert some control over the number of stimuli in the client's clinical environment. If the client is over-whelmed by the number of stimuli and distracted from therapy, the clinician can remove or mask stimuli that might distract the client.

Some objects can be physically removed from the clinic room, such as toys and clinical materials not to be used in that particular therapy session. Other things, such as a wall-mounted mirror, cannot be removed; they can be cov-ered or seating can be arranged in such a way as to reduce their influence. Let us view this means of stimulus manipulation in this way:

▶ S+ −R−R +
8≠ −R−R ≠
8≠ −R−R ≠

Response Manipulation with the CIM

Shaping

Shaping is an operant technique used to create a new behavior—a behavior that the client cannot perform. In shaping, the goal behavior *is not* set forth for the client (this will be added later) and is not part of pure shaping. When shaping is used, any client behavior the clinician feels approximates the goal behavior is rewarded. The principle here is that the reward will increase the likelihood that this behavior will occur again. At the same time, behaviors that do not approximate the goal receive no contingency. This means that those behaviors will extinguish because there is no reward. The process is referred to as *successive approximation*. The technique was developed in experimental work with animals. There is no cognition involved in the process. If the speech clinician uses this technique in its pure form, it is very inefficient. The client does not know what the goal behavior is, and the occurrences of approximated behaviors occur randomly.

Token Economy

The token economy is a special system of providing rewards for a client. One of the problems with giving specific rewards is that clients tend to tire of being given the same reward repeatedly over a period of time. There is also the problem of finding a single reward that is meaningful to a group of clients. The token economy solves these two problems. Tokens are saved by the clients to purchase rewards after therapy or at a specific time that will not interfere with therapy. The token can be anything that the clinician has at hand: pieces of paper, poker chips, or checkers. They are given to the client in place of a specific reward. The tokens themselves become rewarding after the client has actually purchased one of the backup rewards. This reward system allows the clinician to select a number of rewards with different prices and allows the client a choice of rewards. The number of tokens given in the clinical situation is determined by the clinician, as is the price of each item the client can purchase. The clinician will adjust this when or if she finds herself spending too much money on rewards. As with our national economy, inflation will set in, and the prices of the rewards will increase.

Eventually, all token economies must come to an end. The rewards must be withdrawn as the behavior becomes more firmly established. The token reward should be paired with verbal praise during the reign of the token economy. The tokens can then be withdrawn as the verbal praise is maintained. This reduces the influence of the backup reward as the behavior becomes stable.

The token economy has many advantages over a traditional reward program. Some advantages include allowing for a variety of rewards, not interrupting therapy while the client consumes a reward, making it easier for the clinician to administer the initial reward, and administering the same initial reward to all clients in a group setting. Tokens are very powerful rewards, and the token economy is a powerful teaching/learning tool. Consider what would happen if you were given $1 for each minute you were early for work or class.

What about a token economy with older clients? I have used a token economy with clients of all ages. With a 17-year-old client who stuttered, I arranged a token economy in the home where he received a token for controlled fluent speech but lost two tokens each time he talked without his controls. What was his reward? When he collected a certain number of tokens, he could use the family car for a date. Another client, 37 years of age, had two cars. One was a large family station wagon and the other was a foreign sports car. The token economy was set up where his wife would give tokens for the correct behavior and take them away for the incorrect behavior. The tokens were counted each morning and the number of tokens determined whether the client drove the sports car to work or had to drive the station wagon. The client had a lot of avoidance motivation to avoid having to take the station wagon to work. It takes a little imagination and a lot of cooperation to use the token economy with older clients, but if it can be arranged, it is well worth the time and effort. Finally, did the client with the two cars divorce his wife because he had to drive the station wagon? No, he sold it and bought a second sports car. You have to be on your toes to keep ahead of your clients.

Client Motivation and the CIM

Can we assume that all our clients are interested in working on their communication problem? Absolutely not. We might assume a division of clients into two groups—children and adults—but this is not the case. Perhaps a more plausible division might be the reason why they came to us in the first place. Clients come to us either because they want help and are searching it out or because some other person in their environment has made the decision for them. This is not a fool-proof system for sorting those clients who want to work from those who don't, but it is the best that I have been able to come up with. Let us pursue this a bit further. If a client himself wants help with his communication problem, I can assume a degree of approach motivation with which I can work. I can also increase this approach motivation through my reward system in the clinical environment.

But what about the client who is sent to us for therapy? It is not the client's choice to come to us; he is forced to attend therapy. What do we do here? We must attempt to create artificial approach motivation in the clinical environment through our reward system. If we are clever enough, this will suffice in this environment, but we will have to make further adjustments when we try to generalize the behavior to other environments, where we do not have direct control over the reward system. Let us take each of these client types—motivated clients and unmotivated clients—and discuss the clinical ramifications of their attitudes toward therapy.

Clients Seeking Therapy

We can make an assumption that clients who come to us seeking assistance have some interest in therapy. Although we are not faced with creating approach motivation in these clients, we still must maintain it. We can accomplish this through our reward system. However, there is a point in many treatment programs where the client loses his approach motivation. As we get closer to the end of therapy and the new speech behavior is almost perfect, approach motivation wanes. If we cannot find an appropriate reward that will maintain the needed approach motivation, perhaps we can find a penalty that the client wants to avoid. We can then use the client's avoidance motivation as a means of maintaining interest in the therapy.

We can also turn to the significant others in the client's external environment to help us maintain approach and avoidance motivation. But we cannot always count on the assistance of the significant others. We have two alternatives regarding the participation of significant others that we will discuss briefly here and then discuss in more detail in later chapters.

Cooperative Significant Others. When we are lucky enough to have significant others who will become involved and assist our client, we can use them in several ways. The most important way we can use them is to create a support system—that is, to make sure that the significant others understand what the client is working on and provide him with moral support as he is resolving his communication problem. For the client, it is nice to be appreciated, and it is also nice to have significant others acknowledge and reward effort. The significant others must be counseled to reward the client's efforts and support him through understanding and, perhaps, even through direct assistance. With cooperation from significant others, we will be able not only to get the new behavior to occur more rapidly, we will also be able to generalize the new behavior faster.

Uncooperative or absent significant others. The task of maintaining the client's approach motivation is a more difficult task when significant others are uncooperative or absent; in these situations, the only people involved in maintaining the motivation are the clinician and the client. Essentially, the client has no support system. We might be able to compensate for this in some way, such as bringing teachers, nurses, and other people who are involved with the client into the picture, even though they are not truly significant others to the client. If we can get these people to provide moral support and understanding, the task is easier. The rewards provided by these people are very important as a supplement to the direct therapeutic rewards that we are providing. We have a real challenge here, but it is imperative that we maintain the client's interest in therapy. Can we also use avoidance motivation with these surrogate significant others? Yes, but this must be done with caution. Surrogate significant others are not sophisticated clinicians. They will need close supervision in the application of penalty, but if the penalty is administered properly, the client's avoidance motivation will be an important factor. The main problems we face when using a variety of people as a support system are consistency and coordination of their efforts.

Clients Sent for Therapy

This type of client is not limited to children whose parents or teachers feel that therapy is needed. This type could also include adult aphasics, adult stutterers, or any other type of client who does not really see the need for therapy. In some instances, a business will recommend therapy for an employee if they feel that the client does not have the communication skills they deem necessary. In any event, both children and adults are included in the category of clients who really do not have an interest in working on their speech. With this type of client we really have a problem. We must create approach motivation if our treatment is going to be effective. Our alternatives are very limited here, and we will probably not have much success in trying to create interest by talking to the clients, especially younger clients. This does not mean that we should not try approaching the client on a cognitive level. It simply means that we need to supplement this with a reward program that will create approach motivation. Artificial though it may be, if we can create approach motivation to get the reward, we have accomplished our goal of getting the person to learn the new speech behavior.

Like the clients who seek therapy for themselves, clients who are sent to us by others may have decreasing approach motivation as therapy progresses. Again, we may have to create avoidance motivation in the client and use this to maintain interest. We can also use the help of the significant others if they are available.

Cooperative Significant Others. With clients sent for therapy, we need a strong support system and we are fortunate if we have cooperative significant others. The client needs all the support and understanding that the significant others can give him. A meaningful reward program is vitally important in the external environment, especially when we attempt to generalize the new behavior to that environment. The clinician must do some very careful counseling with the significant others so they not only understand the lack of interest on the part of the client, but also how their support and reward system will help the client in therapy. Careful supervision of this support system is vital. The supervision can be in the form of reports from the significant others, but in one way or another, the clinician must be aware of what is transpiring in the external environment.

Uncooperative or Absent Significant Others. If we have any clinical expertise, we need it most when we are faced with a client who has no desire to be in therapy and no one in their environment for support. We can create approach motivation in the clinic room, but the minute the client leaves this environment, there is no support or encouragement from significant others. The best we can do is to enlist the help of other people in the client's environment (teachers, nurses, occupational therapists, physical therapists, and physicians) and make the most of the support that they will give us in providing external rewards for the client. All is not lost in this situation, but our clinical skills will be taxed to the utmost. The use of avoidance motivation through penalty can still be used in this situation, but *extreme* caution must be used, since the other people assisting us in providing penalty are not trained in our specialty. We are still faced with the problems of consistency and coordination of the efforts of people who agree to help us.

C H A P T E R

THE LEARNING ENVIRONMENT

◆ Synopsis

We may now understand the role of the Clinical Interaction Model (CIM) in therapy, but without the client's attention, the CIM is not operational. We can assist the client in focusing and maintaining his attention by creating a clinical environment that is conducive to learning. This learning environment is fundamental to any successful therapy program. With some exceptions, the clinician has control over the clinical environment and can modify it if it is interfering with therapy. This chapter deals with these issues as they relate to therapy.

Attending Behaviors

The most important ingredient for learning is attention. If a student is not attending to lectures in classes, more than likely he is not learning anything. (Of course there are professors who, even if you attend to their lectures, do not teach you anything. But let us hope that this is the exception rather than the rule.) The same principle of attention applies to clients in therapy. If they are not attending to the therapy, they are not going to learn anything from the experience. The clinical process will not work if the client is not attending to therapy. There is an old story that tells about the importance of attention. It goes this way:

A farmer once had a mule that knew how to do tricks. It was a highly trained mule, and the farmer delighted in the fact that he had the only "educated" mule in the county. However, his crops failed one year, and he desperately needed money to pay his debts on his farm. So, he had to face the prospect of selling his mule. Another farmer had heard about the educated mule and made the owner an offer he could not refuse. So the new owner took the mule to his farm, and called in his friends to see the mule's tricks. THE MULE JUST STOOD THERE! He did not do any of his tricks, and all of the new owner's friends had a good laugh about how he had been fooled into thinking the mule could perform tricks. The very angry new owner took the mule back to the original owner and confronted him with the fact that the mule would not perform tricks. The original owner asked the new owner to show him how he went about getting the mule to perform. So, the new owner stood in front of the mule and gave all of the commands for the tricks. Again, the mule just stood there. The original owner's face lit up and he said, "No wonder he won't perform his tricks. You are doing it wrong." With that, the original owner went over to the woodpile and got a 2 × 4 about five feet long. He walked over in front of the mule, and with a hefty swing, he broke it over the mule's head. Then he turned to the new owner and said, "First of all, you have to get his attention."

The moral of the story is you must get the attention of your client before he will learn anything in your therapy. This is the first priority. You must create an environment in your clinic room that is conducive to learning—that is, an environment where the client will attend to you and your therapy rather than attend to some other stimuli in the environment.

Sensory Integration

Human beings have basically five sensory channels for receiving stimuli. We can hear things through the auditory channel, see things through the visual channel, smell things through the olfactory channel, taste things through the gustatory channel, and feel things through the bodily sense channel. I have taken a few liberties with this last channel by combining factors such as kinesthesia, proprioception, and other body senses into a single channel for the sake of clarity. Be aware that this channel receives body sensory information from many sources.

We are under constant bombardment from a multitude of stimuli, which we integrate into a meaningful unit we can deal with in terms of adjustment to our environment. Important stimuli are attended to while unimportant stimuli are evaluated and then ignored. Take just a minute and try to figure out how many stimuli are impinging on you as you read this chapter. Consider the stimuli in your external environment that are attempting to get your attention. If you are in a library (where I have found it impossible to study), you find that there are people walking past you and there is the scraping of chairs as people get up from study tables. If the air conditioning or the heating is not working properly you may be either too cold or too hot. Regardless of where you are, stop reading for a moment and consider the number of potentially distracting stimuli in your environment. But do not get so distracted that you forget to come back to our discussion.

Now, let us consider the things that are going on inside of you—your internal environment—that are acting as stimuli, trying to get your attention. Your ears may still be ringing from the rock concert you went to last night, your head may ache from a cold, your stomach may be upset, your nose may be running from an allergy, or your eyes may hurt from too much reading (a common but unfounded complaint from many of my students). Again, stop reading for a moment and take an inventory of your internal stimuli. If you have all the ailments presented above, do not resume your reading. You are not really learning anything anyway, since you are being distracted by all of these stimuli. Come back to the book when you are feeling better.

Finally, we add to the list internal thoughts, emotions, and feelings that are also vying for your attention. How do we cope with all these factors? How do we attend to any one thing? Humans have the ability to sort out the important stimuli and attend to these, while the other stimuli are placed in the background. Even though we may be attending to one stimulus, if another stimulus is urgent, we will shift our attention to it. You are attending to your reading at this instant, but if you suddenly had a muscle cramp in your leg, your attention would shift to the pain in your leg. Once the pain left, you could shift back to reading.

The Figure–Ground Concept

Figure–ground is a fundamental concept in Gestalt psychology. We have all seen examples of it in basic psychology texts where an illustration shows a white vase against a black background or field. But, as we look at it, we suddenly see the profiles of two faces looking at each other. Now the profiles are black and the background or field is white. What we see depends on what we are focusing our attention. This example concerns only the visual channel, but the same concept applies to all the sensory channels in humans. How many times have you sat in on a less-than-stimulating lecture and found yourself listening to noises out in the hall? Your auditory figure–ground shifted, so that the noises were the figure while the lecture was the ground. Or, perhaps instead of watching the professor draw diagrams on the board, you found yourself looking at the bald spot on his head. These examples illustrate a figure–ground problem within a particular sensory channel.

We can now extend this to figure–ground problems *between channels*. Let us go back to the boring lecture. We would both agree that the auditory channel should be the figure, with all other channels being ground. However, the lecture is just before lunch and you missed breakfast that day. You now find that all your attention is focused on how hungry you are, and the lecture is background. Another example is attempting to study when the television is on: The textbook is very stuffy and you find yourself instead listening to the soap opera.

Clinical Implications

Could the figure–ground relationship possibly influence the transactions between the clinician and the client? Yes, if your client is attending to something other than you and your therapy, you will accomplish very little. You must first get your client's attention like the mule. This means that you, the clinician, must be the figure in the clinic room and determine which sensory channels you are going to use in your teaching. If you are going to produce the sound for the child to imitate, the figure channel you are using is the auditory channel. The visual channel may contribute some information, but the auditory channel is the primary source of information. On the other hand, if you are going to show the client where to place the tongue during the production, the visual channel is the primary source of information.

Your first clinical task is to determine which channel is going to be the figure channel. This will depend on what your clinical task is at the time. Your second task is to determine what the figure will be in the figure channel. Let us consider an example. You decide that the auditory channel is going to be the figure channel. Your task then is to make certain that the other channels are controlled to the extent that they will not interfere with your choice and they do not distract your client. You need to determine if there are visual, olfactory, or bodily sense stimuli in the clinic room that might interfere. (We are not concerning ourselves with the gustatory channel, since it is not a factor in this example.) There always seems to be a mirror in therapy rooms, so you might seat the client in such a way that the reflection in the mirror is not distracting. The seating arrangement could also control the client's likelihood of being distracted by a window in the room. If the room is extremely stuffy, you might open the door for awhile and air out the room before therapy starts. If the room has a shelf of toys that might distract the client, you could cover them with a cloth during therapy. When you control these potentially distracting stimuli, you are creating a learning environment. You are helping the client maintain his attention on you and your therapy.

Once you have the auditory channel as the figure channel, you must determine if there are other auditory stimuli that will interfere with the auditory figure–ground relationship. A clinician might have controlled all of the stimuli in the room that would cause a shift to another figure channel, but still have a problem maintaining the figure–ground relationship within the figure channel she selected. Clinic rooms in the public schools often are rooms that no one else needed or wanted. They are sometimes located right next to the bathrooms, and every time a toilet is flushed so is therapy. Then there is the noise in the hallway. Is outside noise an insurmountable problem? Perhaps in some instances, but if interfering sounds cannot be eliminated they can sometimes be masked by a controlled sound in the clinic room. Once, when working in a clinic room where there was a great deal of distracting noise, I brought a portable radio into the room and tuned it to a local station that played nothing but soft, innocuous music. I turned up the radio to the point where the music masked most of the extraneous noise and found that the client maintained his attention better during therapy. Yes, there are problems in creating and maintaining a learning environment for our clients, but we have already discussed how the clinician should be cognitively involved in the therapy.

Finally, we have the presence of the clinician herself in the clinic room. We will deal with the clinician as a separate entity rather than as a part of the general environment in the clinic room. The clinician can create many problems herself in terms of disturbing the client's figure–ground relationship. During many years of supervision, I have witnessed some interesting problems in this vein. One clinician, attempting to work in the auditory channel, could not get the client to maintain the figure–ground relationship. The client continued to shift to the visual channel. The clinician was wearing earrings made of three successively smaller hoops suspended one within the other. The hoops rotated independently as the earrings themselves swung with each head movement. It was fascinating to watch, not only for the client but also for the supervisor. This might be appropriate for hypnosis, but not speech therapy. Jewelry can be very distracting, particularly for young clients with neurological involvement, where there is already a problem of distractibility. The clinician must take care not to provide distractions in dress, mannerisms, and other behaviors. They are self-defeating.

This concept of figure–ground relationships in the clinic room is shown in Figure 5.1. It should be carefully noted that in this model the client provides constant feedback to the clinician in terms of what he is attending to. The clinician must be attending to the client for this feedback to be of any value. This is part of the monitoring and evaluation that the clinician must do in each succeeding clinical transaction. With my client, Gary (see Chapter 1), I was too involved in attempting to follow my lesson plan to notice that Gary was not paying attention to me. This information was being provided for me, but I was not attending to it. Therefore, I did not make the necessary changes to correct the problem.

Figure 5.1 also shows that the clinician has control over the external environment, that is, the clinic room. She can eliminate visually distracting items from sight by either removing them or masking them. She can also control the seating arrangement to control potentially distracting visual stimuli. Unfortunately, the clinician does not have direct control over the internal environment of the client. If the client is feeling ill or has a headache, this will interfere with therapy by distracting the client. It may be best to terminate the therapy while the client is not feeling good, since little, if anything, is going to be accomplished. However, this decision is dependent on the policy of the agency where the therapy is being provided.

The most pertinent example of the implementation of the figure–ground concept I've experienced in therapy occurred in an agency where, as a clinician, I worked with children who had severe neurological problems. We did therapy with the children in a darkened, sound-treated room with the child placed in a bathtub filled with warm water. The only light in the room was a small flashlight, which was directed at the face of the clinician. In some instances, the clinician would apply bright red lipstick to further call the child's attention to the mouth. When these children were freed of distracting stimuli and were able to concentrate on their clinical tasks, their performance improved dramatically. This was the ultimate in stimulus control. We recognized that this was an artificial environment, and as soon as the children were adjusted to this environment and performing their clinical tasks at a high level of proficiency, other stimuli were gradually introduced. We were careful to present the stimuli at levels below the child's threshold of distractibility. Over a period of time, the children were able to work in a regular clinic room, maintaining their attention on therapy and not being distracted by the various stimuli in the room.

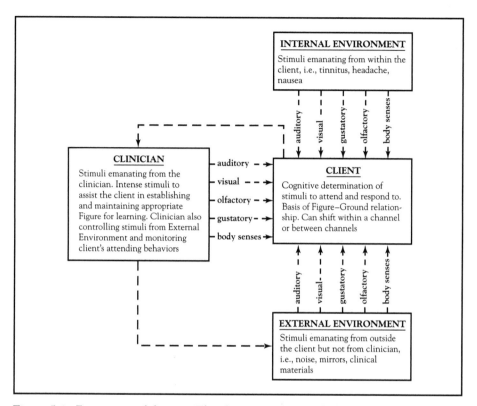

Figure 5.1. Figure–ground diagram. The client receives stimuli through five sensory channels. These stimuli emanate from three sources: his internal environment, his external environment, and the clinician. The client determines which of the numerous stimuli to attend to. This stimulus then becomes the figure which all remaining stimuli become ground. The clinician must compete with other stimuli in order to get the client to attend to therapy. Therapy then becomes the figure and all other stimuli are ground.

If the above example illustrates good use of the figure–ground control, let me give another example and have you analyze it and see what is wrong with the clinical environment. The client in this example is a 16-year-old male with a slight voice quality disorder. The clinic room has a mirror along one wall, a chalkboard on the opposite wall, and a large window on the outside wall. The clinician has arranged the table in the room so that when she is seated for therapy, her back is to the window and the client is facing her across the table. In order to brighten up the rather drab office, she has hung travel posters from Hawaii showing surfing and beach scenes on either side of the mirror and the chalkboard. She has also hung along the top of the chalkboard pictures her younger clients have drawn. The furniture in the room is for younger clients, and the only adult-sized chair she has is the one she uses. She has worn a heavy wool suit to work that day and, being warm, she opens the window a bit, even though it is the middle of winter. She keeps all of her clinical materials on the table in the room, including the stimulus cards for younger clients, toys, pencils, papers, and records.

When she dressed for work that day, she decided to wear the wool suit and gold accessories. She put an intricate pin on the lapel of her suit, and put on a gold charm bracelet and dangling earrings. She finished this off with three large gold rings, two on her right hand. She did her fingernails that day with a very bright red polish in order to set off the gold rings. The glasses she decided to wear had rhinestones in the frames, and she had her initials engraved in the lower left-hand corner of the left lens. The last thing she did before leaving for work was to splash on a generous dose of perfume.

I am sure that if you carefully study this example, you might find a few things that could interfere with the therapy interaction. This is, perhaps, an outlandish example, but how many of these things have you seen occurring in therapy you have observed? (We are applying the OP Rule [other people] again.)

We have gone from one extreme to another in terms of the clinical environment, but before we leave this topic we should deal with some practical problems in the clinic room. Let me give you an example of one such problem. The clinician I was observing was working with a 4-year-old child. The clinic room was furnished with two adult-sized chairs, two small chairs for children, and a table to hold the clinical materials. The therapy started with both the clinician, and the child seated in the small chairs. Therapy was progressing nicely and the child was attending to all of the clinical activities. However, the clinician had some difficulty working with the materials on the table since she was sitting so low. She was also a bit uncomfortable sitting on such a small chair. She solved the problems by moving to an adult chair while the child remained in the small chair. The clinician could now use the materials on the table more easily and she was comfortable in the larger chair. This arrangement soon created other problems. The clinician now had to look down on the child since she was sitting so much higher. Further, since it was now easier to use the materials on the table, she made extensive use of them, but the child was sitting so low he had trouble seeing what was happening. There was an obvious answer to all of this; place the child in an adult chair. This again placed the clinician and the child at about the same height, and the child was now able to see the materials on the table. Things went fine for about 3 minutes, and then the clinician began to lose the child's attention. He began to wiggle in the chair, swing his feet back and forth, and behave in a very restless fashion. The clinician tried to get his attention back on therapy by increasing the rewards, but was not successful. The remainder of the therapy session was not at all productive. The clinician was baffled, since this was not typical behavior for this child.

During our conference on the therapy session I pointed out two possible explanations for this behavior. The most plausible one had to do with sitting in a chair where the feet do not touch the floor. This is very uncomfortable, and the client's legs have a tendency to "go to sleep." The child's figure–ground relationship had shifted from attending to therapy to attending to the discomfort in his legs. He was wiggling and swinging his legs in order to prevent gangrene from setting in. If someone in the therapy session had to be uncomfortable, it should have been the clinician. She would be creating a comfortable learning environment for the child, not herself.

There is still another possible explanation for the behavior of this child. This type of behavior is often seen in children who need to go to the toilet. Younger children may not ask if they may go to the toilet. They just wiggle more and more. They are obviously attending more to their bodily need than to therapy. More than one clinician has ignored these behavioral signs of impending disaster and had to clean up the clinic room. If in doubt, just ask. An ounce of prevention is worth a pound of paper toweling.

We mentioned clinical materials in earlier examples, but now let us be a bit more specific. Many speech clinicians going to a therapy session resemble a bag lady. If you are not familiar with the term, it is used to describe women who carry all their earthly possessions with them in a shopping bag. The therapist takes her bag of materials into the clinic room and proceeds to lay out all the materials for the session on the table. She must have a game, a toy, or an instrument for every moment of therapy. There is no imagination evident in the therapy planning, just a dependence on gimmicks. The last thing the therapist takes out of the bag is a tape recorder, so that she can record her therapy session (I wonder if these clinicians ever listen to their therapy). The table is now all but covered with games, books, pictures, toys, and the tape recorder. The clinician then brings the child into the clinic room and wonders why the child is not attending to therapy. The materials should have been left in the bag and the bag kept under the table. The tape recorder, if actually necessary, should be placed out of the child's direct line of vision, perhaps at the far end of the table. It might also be covered with a piece of cloth to mask it. There is nothing more distracting than clutter in a clinic room. Whatever happened to the speech clinician who could go into therapy with nothing more than a pencil and paper and motivate her clients?

Then there are mirrors. Every clinic room must have a mirror. The really good ones take up an entire wall. These large mirrors give the child twice as much to look at. And clinicians usually have the seating arranged in such a way that the mirror is either directly in front of the child or to one side of him.

They may not be using the mirror as part of the therapy, but the mirror is still there. Would it not make more sense to arrange the seating so the mirror was not in the child's line of vision, perhaps with the mirror behind the child? If the mirror is needed for a segment of therapy, it is simply a matter of turning a chair around.

Mirrors take on added horror when they are one-way mirrors. These mirrors work fine until someone turns on a light in the observation room. You now have a window between the rooms. When the child sees other people watching him and then the light goes out and the window is a mirror again, you have a very distracted child. In one instance where this occurred, the child had to be moved to another clinic room where there was no mirror, and finding one was no mean task. When the child saw the fleeting images of people in the mirror (when the light was turned on briefly), he thought they were ghosts and that was the end of therapy in that room.

If you are working with a highly distractible child, you should attempt to reduce the stimuli in your room as described earlier. You can also arrange the seating in such a way that the distractions in the room are minimized. You can place your chair in a corner of the room where there are no distracting stimuli behind you and place the child's chair facing you. In this way, the child has nothing to look at but you. This is a simple but effective way to control the child's attention.

One of the most ingenious devices you can use to work with a highly distractible client is the *pinhole mask*. This is simply a mask that you place over the client's eyes where he can only see out of two small pinholes. This serves to reduce the scope of the visual field. I saw this demonstrated with some severely involved children with cerebral palsy, and the effect it had on their coordination was startling. A severely involved athetoid who could barely walk due to head movements triggered by various stimuli in his visual field walked almost normally when wearing such a mask. With another client, whose head movements triggered a series of reflexes that resulted in his falling out of his wheelchair, the pinhole mask eliminated the reflex chain and made it possible for him to receive therapy.

Before we leave the topic, we must consider the effect that group therapy will have on the learning environment. As we add clients to the clinical environment, we are adding potentially distracting stimuli. This is an extremely important factor that we must consider when setting up group therapy. Some of our clients, because of age, maturity, type of disorder, or some other factor, may not be able to tolerate this increase in stimuli. There are no hard and fast rules to apply here. This is a clinical judgment that the speech clinician must make. She may decide that a certain client can tolerate the group setting, but then find that the client cannot learn in such a setting. She may be able to modify the group setting in such a way that the client can operate satisfactorily. If not, she will have to make some arrangements to provide the client with individual attention. (The group therapy process is discussed in detail in Chapter 10.)

Your challenge, as a speech clinician, is to create and maintain a clinical environment that is conducive to learning. Give your clients some assistance in maintaining their attention to your therapy. Make your therapy interesting; show some enthusiasm. People pay attention to things that are interesting and entertaining. Therapy does not have to be boring. The only person who can make therapy boring is the clinician. Is it unprofessional to have fun in therapy, to enjoy therapy? Let us keep in mind that awful therapy creates many problems in figure–ground relationships. The client is confused. He often does not know which channel to attend to. And when he does know and attempts to attend to the figure channel, it is so boring and confusing he begins to attend to other channels. Think of your therapy as a television program and your client as the one who controls the remote control for his television set. If your program is the best available, he will tune you in. However, if there is something better on another channel, he will tune to it, and you will have lost him. I have seen some therapy where I certainly understood why the client tuned his set to commercials, since they were more interesting.

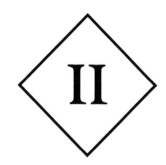
THE *HOW* OF THERAPY

CHAPTER

6

EVALUATION AND PLANNING

◆ Synopsis

*Client evaluation and therapy planning are the foundation of therapy.
Without correct identification of the problem, appropriate therapy cannot be
planned. Further, if the communication problem is classified incorrectly, it
leads to the application of incorrect therapy. Careful examination of the
client will lead to a correct diagnosis, and this is the basis of an appropriate
therapy plan. The vehicle for the evaluation and planning phase of therapy
is the Clinical Interaction Model (CIM). The three functions of the CIM
in this initial phase of therapy are data gathering, data processing, and data
sharing. The data gathered are used to build data banks about the client and
his disorder. Associated data banks are also used in data processing as we
determine the diagnosis of the client. All data banks are used when we share
the data with the client in the final planning conference.*

Recognizing the many variations in evaluation and planning procedures, I
will present a generic organization that you can then adapt to your unique
clinical environment. The steps involved are (1) interviewing the client and
taking a case history; (2) directly examining the client, including the administration of diagnostic tests to determine the type and severity of the disorder;
(3) integrating and synthesizing all data to determine the exact type of disorder, its description, its severity, and an appropriate treatment program; and

(4) conferencing with the client or the significant other to discuss the findings and proposed treatment program.

In Chapter 3, the three main functions of the CIM were listed as gathering information, teaching, and sharing information. It was also pointed out that the CIM had some special functions in the evaluation and planning phase of the clinical process. These special functions are extensions of the data gathering and data sharing functions and the application of the CIM to the clinician's cognitive evaluation of the information gathered in the evaluation and planning process.

Since the evaluation and planning process is essentially data based, we will view the roles of the CIM in this phase of therapy as (1) data gathering, (2) data processing, and (3) data sharing. Instead of discussing each step of the evaluation and planning process as a separate entity, we will discuss the steps as they relate to the data gathering, data processing, and data sharing roles of the CIM.

The Role of the CIM in Data Gathering

The purpose of the data gathering procedure is to build a database—a grouping of information related to a concept or an entity. For example, our database of articulation disorders contains all the information we have about communication problems associated with articulation. Associated with this data base are our other data bases concerning phonetics, anatomy and physiology, neurology, acoustics, and so forth. We continue to build data bases even after completing our training program, adding more information to existing data bases and developing new ones.

The database we build for a client contains all the pertinent information we have collected about the client. This database, along with all associated data bases, provides us with the information necessary to make our diagnosis of the client's disorder and plan an appropriate treatment program. Our first step in the evaluation and planning process is data gathering in order to build a client database.

We gather information from many sources, but regardless of the source, the information comes to us mainly in two forms: auditory and visual. Each contributes to our overall understanding of the problem we are assessing.

The main source of auditory data is the client's responses to direct questions both during the informal interview and during the formal case history. Other auditory data are available through the client's attempts to perform speech tasks requested by the clinician. The clinician may model a particular sound and have the client attempt to imitate the production. The errors the client makes provide us with important information regarding the classification and etiology of the disorder and help us plan a treatment program.

Motor skills are best evaluated by visual inspection. Motor skills are manifested by the client's production of requested motor movements, such as diadochokinetic sequences or the production of specific sounds. Visual examination also includes the aesthetics of speech production. For example, a sound may be produced acoustically correct but physiologically incorrect, such as producing the [f] sound with the upper lip contacting the lower teeth.

Interview/Case History

The interview/case history is your first contact with the client and, if involved, his significant others. This is where you make your first clinical impression; you either impress them positively with your professionalism or negatively with your lack thereof. You are judged by your demeanor. Do you give the impression of being knowledgeable, professional, friendly, understanding, and empathic? Are you the person the client or his significant others would trust with the treatment of the communication disorder?

In their 1989 text, *The Clinical Interview: Using DSM–III–R*, Othmer and Othmer include a chapter, "Strategies for Rapport," that will assist you with your evaluation and planning procedures. They list six specific aspects of good technique: putting the client and yourself at ease; expressing compassion; evaluating the patient's insight; showing your expertise to the patient; establishing yourself as an authority; and balancing these roles in therapy. I recommend that you explore their text.

The clinician's main activity during the interview/case history is asking questions. Your stimulus in the CIM is asking questions or attempting to get the client to expand on a point. Design your questions so they help you learn about the client and his environments—what may have caused the disorder, what treatment he has had in the past, and so forth. In all probability, you will go into the interview with some preconceived notions about the client. For example, if the client was referred to you, the referral form will tell you something about the probable communication disorder. In these situations, focus your questions on confirming or denying this information. Throughout the interview, try to find a series of factors or events that, when taken together, form an etiology that might explain the client's disorder. If you can find the etiology, it will confirm your tentative classification of the disorder; you must then confirm this classification in your diagnostic examination.

The CIM is central to the interactions during the initial interview. In these transactions, the stimulus is that question, and the response that you evaluate is the client's answer to your question. In addition to listening carefully to the responses, you observe carefully to make certain your questions were understood. You will also be observing the communication disorder and forming your initial impressions. By the end of the interview and case history, you should have a general classification of the disorder in mind and some insights into its severity.

Examination of the Client

In some instances, you may feel this step is not necessary because the disorder was so obvious during the interview and case history. However, even though you may think you have classified the disorder, you need to verify the classification through formal and informal testing. You should have an opinion of the classification of the disorder before this examination; you cannot select appropriate testing materials unless you have a classification for the disorder. An illustration of this situation is presented in the clinical example found at the end of this chapter.

The CIM is again the vehicle used for exploration. You will prompt more speech from the client for your analysis. You will ask specific questions to ferret out clues about the disorder. You will do some informal testing of various disorders, if for no other reason than just to eliminate them from consideration. Each of these transactions is a means of gathering data and of testing a hypothesis. As you complete each transaction, you carefully plan where the next transaction should go. You are deeply involved cognitively in the CIM, listening and watching the client, evaluating what he is telling you, putting the information into your data base, and planning where the next transaction should go. It is like playing a detective game where you gather clues and try to find the guilty person. False leads are rejected while meaningful clues provide you with an indication of the direction you should go in your pursuit of the answer. You build a database during these transactions that will eventually provide you with an answer. You are cognitively, deeply involved in each transaction, weighing each response against your basic knowledge (database) of each disorder. As more pertinent information is uncovered, you will focus your questions and informal testing more directly on a specific disorder. And it is through this process of inquiry and observation that you finally reach your diagnosis of the disorder. Once this is determined you can move on to more in-depth testing.

Diagnostic Testing

Once the disorder has been tentatively classified, appropriate tests can be selected to evaluate the disorder more thoroughly and to verify or refute the diagnosis. The tests you give are to support or reject your clinical hypothesis regarding the classification of the disorder. If the tests support your hypothesis, you can assume your classification is correct. If the tests fail to support the hypothesis, you must rethink your classification, form another hypothesis, and go through the testing process again. You continue this process until you can explain why the incorrect communication behaviors occur.

The various tests are administered through the CIM. You provide the stimulus according to each test's rules of administration. You then evaluate the client's responses, again in accordance with a particular test's guidelines. Cognitively, you are evaluating the responses as the client gives them and entering the responses on the data sheets provided with the test. You are building a data base for later decisions. In addition to tests directed to the specific disorder, you will test other factors that you deem important, such as intelligence, auditory acuity, and so forth.

The Role of the CIM in Data Processing

The most important thing to recognize here is that the data collection and data processing procedures are not mutually exclusive. Even as the data gathering process proceeds and the database is expanding, we are processing the data and reaching tentative conclusions. These are the initial, general diagnoses we make and test, seeking out the correct direction to proceed with the evaluation. These early diagnoses are our attempts to focus more closely on the actual diagnosis. The closer we get to the completion of the data gathering, the more data processing we are involved in. When does the process shift completely to data processing? There is probably no complete shift, only a shift in emphasis since we will be gathering additional information throughout the evaluation and planning process.

After we have gathered all the data we feel is necessary, we must synthesize it before we can reach a conclusion regarding the type of disorder, its severity, and any unique feature associated with it. As we review the data and compare it with our various data banks, we are trying to find the "best fit," to find the most agreement between our client data base and the various disorder databases. Each time we compare our client's data bank with related data banks, we are testing a hypothetical diagnosis. And when we are not satisfied with the fit, we must formulate another hypothetical diagnosis.

We are now at that stage of the process where we begin to talk to ourselves. (Everybody does this from time to time. Sometimes it seems like this is the only way we can talk to someone as intelligent as we are!) Interact with yourself in determining the proper diagnosis of the client's communication disorder, but I recommend that you not do this verbally where others might observe you. You could find yourself being referred to another clinic for another type of diagnostic procedure.

However, talking to yourself is not a negative or strange behavior. I find that when I am deeply into a theoretic or abstract issue, I sort through the issue better if I verbalize it to myself and talk it out. This is an important means of problem solving for me. I simply do not allow others to watch this somewhat schizophrenic interaction. I also find I can tolerate severe criticism from myself when I might reject it from someone else. The CIM will assist you in getting this constructive problem-solving conversation started with yourself.

The CIM now applies to us as we talk among ourselves about how well our data fit various data banks we are considering, what variables we need to consider, what the possible cause of the disorder might be, and so forth. You may even be arguing with yourself at this point. The end result will be a carefully thought-out diagnosis.

As you consider various diagnostic classifications, there is a possibility that no "best fit" satisfies you. If this occurs, you will have to go back to data gathering and further expand your client's database. You cannot complete the data processing step until you have reached a diagnosis that you are comfortable with, a diagnosis that has a "best fit" with not only the client's data base but also the associated data bases you are considering.

When you have the correct diagnosis of the client's communication disorder, you are halfway through the data processing step. The diagnosis gives you only a general idea of what the disorder is. For example, let us imagine that we have just had a child referred to us and the only information on the referral form is that the child has an articulation disorder. All we know at this point is that the child has some problems associated with the production of phonemes. We do not know which phonemes are involved or if the problem is a sound substitution, sound distortion, sound omission, or the addition of sounds. We do not have enough information to discuss the client with anyone or even to think about designing a treatment program.

The necessary second half of the diagnostic step is a detailed description of the client's disorder. This information comes from the client examination and the diagnostic tests we give, but it needs to be synthesized into a descriptive behavior profile. We can say a client is a stutterer, but then we have to describe the stuttering. We add the statement that the stuttering is severe (this reflects how we as listeners react to the stuttering and has no relevance as to how the stutterer views his stuttering). This is still much too vague. To make the data meaningful, we must add information about the average duration of the stuttering blocks, the number of blocks in a given time period, and the number and types of secondary mannerisms the client has. The picture is getting more complete now and is almost ready for us to use as a base to plan therapy. Once we add a report on the client's attitudes and beliefs about his stuttering, our diagnosis is complete.

We have the general classification of the disorder, a detailed description of how the disorder manifests itself, and a record of the client's attitudes about therapy. We are now ready to plan a therapy program. Review the information you received in the interview/case history and the diagnostic examination in order to plan therapy. Then, review the client's data base for any factors that could negatively influence therapy, such as hearing loss or mental retardation. This broad data base is then used to plan therapy for the client's particular communication disorder. Although it is not necessary to plan the details of the program at this time, the short- and long-term goals, as well as some sort of prognosis, should be thought through as you plan your therapy. You must have a general treatment plan to present to the client and/or the significant others when you finish your evaluations.

The Role of the CIM in Data Sharing

It is now time to have the final conference with the client and/or significant others. We again turn to the CIM. You will be providing the stimulus in this environment, giving facts and details, providing a diagnostic classification of the communication disorder, and setting forth a treatment program along with some sort of a prognosis. In order to make certain your information is being received and understood, carefully observe reactions to what you are saying and invite questions.

The final conference is an important interaction between you and the client and/or the significant others. This is where you finalize your relationship with the client and establish a cooperative relationship with the significant others. This is also where you establish your credibility as a professional. The foundations of your relationships among yourself, your clients, and their significant others are dependent on your professional behavior in this situation. The next step in your clinical process is direct therapy with the client in the therapy room.

Clinical Example

The evaluation/planning step in the clinical process is ideal for demonstrating the level of cognitive involvement the clinician has in therapy. It is much like a game of *Clue*, where players have to find the guilty party. In this step, we have to gather information from many sources, cognitively process it, come to some tentative conclusions, argue with ourselves, reevaluate our findings, test our conclusions, and finally make our deduction as to what the "guilty party" is. And then, knowing the guilty party, we need to set forth a means of dealing with it and rectifying the "crime."

Rather than create an example of a diagnostic evaluation, I have taken an actual case where the diagnosis presented some unique challenges. As you read this, consider how the CIM is used (1) in data gathering, (2) in data processing, and (3) in data sharing.

In this part of the evaluation, the CIM is used as a means of gathering information and building the client data base. Initially, the data gathering is quite informal and conversational and is used primarily to establish rapport. Once this is achieved, the conversation becomes more formal, with questions directed toward the client's history. The following general rules apply to the role of the clinician in the transactions.

- *Clinician's stimulus:* The clinician's stimulus consists mainly of asking general questions to establish rapport and specific questions to collect data for the clinical history.

- *Clinician's cognitions:* Cognitions focus on both what the client is saying and how he is saying it, attending to the appropriateness of the client's responses as well as the information contained in them. They also focus on monitoring the client's attention during the interaction and gathering information on the client's history and on speech and language behaviors.

- *Clinician's response:* The response is not the main focus of the transaction and mainly takes the form of responding appropriately to what the client has said before moving to the next question.

The Evaluation/Planning Process

Our client is a 33-year-old female nurse. She was referred to us by a hospital clinic as a severe stutterer. The referral indicated she had been at two clinics prior to the referring clinic. Each clinic had referred her, stating that the problem was too severe for the services offered by their program.

When the client presents herself for the diagnostic evaluation, we understand why the other clinics had referred her to still more clinics; she presents the most bizarre speech patterns we have ever seen. Initially, we carry on a casual conversation with the client to establish rapport. However, when we start the collection of data through a case history, we use the CIM in a more formal way. We are now more cognitively involved, processing the information she is giving us and observing the nonverbal behaviors associated with her speech. We note that every syllable of her speech is labored, as she pounds her legs, bends over so far her head is between her knees, runs out of breath and gasps for air, contorts her face into severe grimaces, twists her head around, shuts her eyes tightly, and so forth. It takes her 2 or 3 minutes to complete even short sentences. She carries a pad and pencil with her and often writes answers instead of speaking.

Our first task is to establish a client database, gathering as much information as we can about the client and the disorder. As we collect information in the interview/case history with the client, we talk to ourselves about what we are finding. Our internal CIM is either supporting or rejecting our early impressions of the client's problem. All data is under scrutiny and related to the impressions we have about the client and the disorder. We also begin to bring into play related databases.

As we observe the client and process the information we have gathered, we find some discrepancy between the diagnosis of stuttering and the speech we are observing. We observe the client struggling to put the tongue to the alveolar ridge to say the [l] sound in the word "look." The distorted movement is not repetitive, but rather a clumsy attempt to place the tongue on the alveolar ridge. She is unable to complete the word because she cannot get her tongue up to the alveolar ridge to say the initial sound. The interruptions in speech do not resemble those of other stutterers we have seen.

In taking the case history, which is long and tedious because of the labored speech, we learn that the client has a history of seizures. When she was in her early teens, she had a long series of grand mal seizures after having meningitis. She was on seizure control medication for 10 years and then voluntarily stopped taking it. There had been no reoccurrence of the seizures for another 10 years, until 3 months ago when they began again. She was having approximately 10 seizures per day and had been put back on her medication. With the reoccurrence of the seizures, her speech was affected and she was referred to a hospital clinic for treatment. She was diagnosed as a stutterer and referred to another clinic. The second clinic confirmed the diagnosis and referred her to a third clinic; the third clinic referred her to us.

As we talk among ourselves, we begin to consider the possibility that the communication disorder is not developmental stuttering but rather neurological stuttering. We review the new information on the seizures and make a new classification. The data we had supported the new classification, so we formed a new hypothesis. This became our new hypothesis: The client is a stutterer, with the strong possibility that the stuttering is neurologically based.

> We still gather information, seeking to confirm or deny our hypothesis. We are now at the stage of testing a number of hypotheses, and we must test each one. Many related databases are called into play. We review the databases of each disorder's classification and then how they agree with the client database. We ask questions to prompt specific behaviors and we observe reactions to the occurrence of the disorder. We are deeply, cognitively involved as we try to find a classification that would explain all the characteristics of the disorder we are observing. We have not yet found a "best fit."

Our task now is to test for the presence of neurological stuttering. We engage our client in a lengthy conversation, observing her speech very carefully. We note two very important speech behaviors our client displays that do not fit the description of neurological stuttering. First, there is the form of stuttering: Neurological stuttering is characterized by rapid and rhythmical repetitions on almost every syllable, but rapid and rhythmical repetitions are not characteristic of our client. The second factor is the absence of a symptom called *La Belle Indifference*. The person who has neurological, or even hysterical, stuttering is not disturbed by it. In fact, for the most part, they seem oblivious to it, and there is no struggle with the stuttering. *La Belle Indifference* is not part of the character of our case. The organic and hysterical factors as a base to our client's stuttering are now very suspect.

> We are deeply into our internal CIM. We keep questioning our classifications of the disorder, and we finally find ourselves questioning the diagnosis on the referral itself. We are now considering changing the disorder type because we have ruled out all variations of the disorder. We are arguing with ourselves, questioning our decisions, our conclusions, the direction of our evaluation. We need to do some specific testing to provide ourselves with new stimuli. No longer do we just ask questions, but we also ask the client to perform certain tasks.

Having essentially ruled out neurological and hysterical stuttering, we must now see if we can verify the general classification of stuttering. The only other classification of stuttering is developmental, and this is highly suspect because of the sudden onset of the stuttering or stuttering-like speech. We decide to do several informal tests to see if we can verify the stuttering classification. The CIM is still in the data gathering mode and is now concerned with the evaluation of a series of behaviors the client is requested to perform. First, we test to see if the client demonstrates the *adaptation effect*, stuttering less and less with successive readings of the same materials. The successive readings result in no decrease in stuttering and even, perhaps, more stuttering. We then try unison reading, reading a short passage with her. Developmental stuttering should all but disappear under this condition, but it has no effect on her speech. We then try a distraction, having her beat time with her hand and speak on the beat. Again, this should decrease the frequency of stuttering, but it has no effect. Finally, we try having her sing. We choose the song "Happy Birthday" since it is a common song, and she says she knows it very well. We would expect the stuttering to diminish if her condition is truly stuttering. The stuttering was altered slightly but did not disappear.

We are now at a pivotal point in our evaluation. We turn to our internal CIM and assess where we are in the evaluation. We have essentially ruled out the organic and hysterical stuttering classification, since the characteristics of the client's stuttering do not resemble behaviors associated with those forms of stuttering. We have also ruled out the developmental classification of stuttering, since not only does the speech pattern not resemble developmental stuttering, but tests of stuttering all proved negative. We must reject the classification of stuttering and search for another disorder type. To do this, we need to gather more data and do some further testing and observing. As we gather the additional data, we are seeking a pattern or some other clue as to what classification we can turn to. It's time to go back to data gathering and the expansion of the client's data base.

Since the client was unable to say the word "look" because of problems with the production of the initial sound, we remove the language element and focus on the motor movement of the sound. We ask the client to make an isolated [l] sound. The client struggles to get the tongue into the proper position, and the voicing is sporadic and delayed. When voicing is produced, it is produced on residual air, and the client is doubled over trying to force out enough air to maintain the sound for even a second. Our internal CIM, processing this information, indicates that voicing is a problem, so we shift our attention to the level of vocalization.

We ask the client to produce an "ah." The voicing is difficult for the client to initiate, and it is sporadic, alternating with exhalation. We begin to talk to ourselves again. Could it be she is stuttering on vocalization? What about the fact that she was having a lot of difficulty initiating the voicing because she could not start the exhalation to introduce the sound? Did we detect that she was having difficulty inhaling enough air to produce the vocalizations and that all her attempts to vocalize were on residual air?

The result of the action of the internal CIM is the establishment of another hypothesis that needs to be tested. Looking for different behaviors, we again test the hypothesis by requesting that the client perform certain tasks, as we watch carefully for behaviors characteristic of the new potential classification, a respiratory disorder. Careful observation indicates that she has very shallow breathing, obviously not deep enough to sustain a vocalization. When instructed to take a deep breath, she attempts to do so but is unable to accomplish it. She is able to perform vegetative breathing but cannot vary from it.

It is time to create a new classification for the disorder. We review what information we have at this point in our evaluation.

1. There is neurological involvement evidenced by the seizures.
2. The classification of stuttering is ruled out.
3. The client has difficulty in moving the articulators to appropriate positions.
4. The client has difficulty in moving the vocal folds to approximation to produce voice.
5. The client has difficulty in shifting from vegetative breathing to voluntary inhalation.

We have a client with a long history of neurological dysfunction, a client who cannot initiate voluntary movements of articulation, vocalization, or respiration. We think this through and decide on a new classification: apraxia. Apraxia is associated with neurological dysfunction and manifests itself in the inability of the client to perform voluntary motor acts while reflexive movements remain functional. We then think of how we can test this new hypothesis. We know that the voluntary movements of the speech mechanisms, the phonatory system, and the respiratory system are impaired, so we need to test the reflexive aspects of the behaviors.

To test the functions of the oral structures, we bring in some food for the client to eat. All of her chewing, sucking, and swallowing activities are normal. To test the vocal function, we get her to laugh, and we listen carefully to her reflexive sounds, such as sighs. Both the laughing and the reflexive sounds are normal. In order to test the respiration, we must get a reflexive inhalation to occur. To cause this we use the client's startle reflex. During a quiet moment in the examination room, we suddenly slam a book on the desk, making a loud and unexpected noise. The client gasps with a sudden air intake. So far our test results support the classification of apraxia involving motor movements of articulation, phonation, and respiration.

Things are going well, and we are certain we are on the right track in viewing the disorder as apraxia. However, in our internal CIM, we question the classification. Does apraxia ever occur in isolation, or is it always associated with other disorders? The internal CIM concludes that there should be an associated aphasia. If there is an aphasia, it would confirm the classification of apraxia. Thus far in the examination, we have not detected any signs of aphasia; so if it is present, it must be a very mild form. We review what we have observed of the client's language functions in our interactions. The only thing that comes to mind is that she periodically gets a quizzical look on her face after we tell or ask her something, and she fails to respond. When we repeat it, perhaps twice, her expression changes to a smile, and she responds appropriately.

We ask the client if she has any difficulty remembering words when answering specific questions. She tells us she cannot recall her telephone number, her address, the names of her children, or other pertinent data about herself. This was information we collected earlier when she used documents such as her driver's license to assist her in answering our questions. We viewed this as a manifestation of stuttering at the time.

When asked about the times she has the quizzical look on her face when we tell her something, she responds that occasionally when people talk to her it sounds like they are speaking a foreign language and that it takes time for her to sort through what she is told until it finally makes sense.

We now have the evidence to support our hypothesis that the client's speech disorder is due to a diffuse apraxia accompanied by a slight receptive and expressive aphasia. With the classification determined, a therapy program can be planned.

> We plan a general approach to the problem and are then ready to talk to the client about our findings and recommendations. We now shift the CIM to data sharing. In this mode, we will tell the client our findings. Then, reversing the CIM, we respond to the client's questions.

With the classification firm in our mind, we have a conference with the client to explain our findings and make recommendations for therapy. We explain how we tested each hypothesis and what our conclusions were. We then explain what apraxia and aphasia are and how we tested and verified that this is the problem. When we invite questions, the client has many questions about the apraxia and the aphasia. She is also concerned about the outcome of therapy and if she can go back to work. We answer these questions to the best of our ability.

> In the final step of the evaluation, we shift the CIM into a teaching mode and demonstrate the therapy techniques to the client. We want her to understand how she will go about relearning how to perform behavior on a voluntary basis. We are not actually teaching new behaviors since the behaviors are still being performed on a reflexive level. This is an important difference in our therapeutic approach, and we explain this carefully to the client. We explain that we will be teaching her how to voluntarily perform behaviors that now only occur on a reflex basis. The therapy is demonstrated to show how we will be operating in therapy and also to show that she can learn to perform the behaviors. This is for the client's morale and motivation.
>
> During the actual therapy sessions, the CIM was usually in the teaching mode, although there were times in almost every therapy session where more data gathering was necessary. This was particularly important when the client had to report on her outside work on breathing, vocalizing, and movements of the articulators. Sharing through the CIM was important, as the clinician shared with the client how well she was doing in therapy. This was one of the main sources of motivation for the client.

We discuss the treatment program and then, with the CIM in the teaching mode, demonstrate how we will teach her to produce the reflexive behaviors on a voluntary basis. The client experiences some limited success and therapy appointments are then scheduled. This brings to a close the evaluation/planning period of therapy.

The evaluation/planning process described above involved a total of four clinical sessions, each lasting 45 minutes. Sixteen treatment sessions were necessary to complete the treatment program, at which time the client was dismissed with complete recovery of all functions. Follow-up was continued for 1½ years with no reoccurrence of any problem. The client went back to work as a nurse and has appeared in a television commercial for a drugstore chain.

CHAPTER

GETTING THE NEW BEHAVIOR TO OCCUR

◆ Synopsis

As we start our therapy, we concentrate on getting a new behavior to occur. The evaluation has been completed, and we have decided on what our behavior change goal is. Our therapy plan has been formed and factors that might interfere with our therapy, such as a hearing loss or dysarthria, have been accounted for. We are now ready to introduce our client to the new behavior we plan to teach. This chapter discusses how the Clinical Interaction Model (CIM) is involved in getting the new behavior to occur.

Antecedent and Contingent Events in the CIM

The focus in this phase of the clinical process is on the contingent events, the reward (R+) and penalty (P). We will use these contingent events to provide approach motivation and avoidance motivation for our clients. The consequences for the attempts by the client to produce the new speech behavior can both encourage the new behavior to occur, R+, or discourage the production of the original error, P. P is very important because the client succeeds in avoiding the penalty by performing the correct behavior. This is a very strong form of reward for the correct behavior. This is not to say that antecedent events are not important. We provide modeling, guidance, and information for the client, all of which are antecedent to the client's attempt to produce the new behavior. We then fade these events as the new behavior is learned.

We must also consider when the behavior we are working with is not a totally new behavior for the client. Perhaps we are working with a client who can produce the [g] in the initial position in a word but distorts it in all other positions. In this case we should view the new behavior not as the production of the [g] sound itself, but as the production of the correct [g] in medial and final positions of words. Fluency is not a new behavior for the stutterer. There are many times when the stutterer is completely fluent. We must get the client to the point where he can create fluent speech when he needs it in difficult speaking situations.

It is during this phase of the clinical process that our clients are faced with their first major learning task. This is where they are going to "learn how to learn." We are emphasizing the contingent events (R+ and P) because they provide the basis of learning; that is, we are attending to therapy as well as the client's approach and avoidance motivation. We will be using ALL of the techniques and procedures we discussed in Chapter 3, but we will combine them into an effective and efficient clinical approach.

Combining Techniques and Procedures

As we begin to combine the teaching techniques and procedures discussed in Chapter 3, we will gradually develop a more efficient and effective clinical approach. We start our therapy with the shaping procedure. A clinical example will help illustrate this point. We then add other techniques and processes, discussing how each addition has influenced therapy with a specific client.

Shaping

The speech clinician has determined that the client has a defective [s] sound. She talks with the client and when an [s] sound occurs that more closely approximates the correct production, she rewards it. She does not tell the client why he is receiving the reward; it is just given. This is shaping in its purest form. However, this type of clinical activity could take years before the [s] is correct in all contexts. The client would probably outgrow it before the clinician corrected it. This does not mean that shaping through successive approximation is not a valuable technique. It only means that we need to make the process more efficient. Let us add modeling to our procedure.

Modeling

After the clinician has determined that the [s] is defective but before the client attempts to produce the sound, the clinician demonstrates the correct production for him. She produces the [s] sound in isolation and tells the client that this is his goal, to produce the sound as she made it for him. Now the client knows what the behavior change goal is, and the clinician can now proceed with shaping through successive approximation. With each attempt that is closer to the correct production, the clinician rewards him and then provides the model again. Our therapy is more efficient now, but we can make it still more efficient by adding other techniques.

Guidance

After the clinician in our example has modeled the [s] sound for the client and has rewarded him for better productions, she reaches a point where the sound is not improving. The client is holding his lower lip too high, and this is distorting the sound slightly. She might then say, "When you make the sound this time, I am going to hold your lower lip down to where it should be when you make the [s] sound. Now listen to it again—[s]." When the client makes his next attempt, the clinician holds the lower lip down slightly to improve the sound production. This is physical guidance. She is guiding him to improve the production of the sound. Our therapy is becoming more efficient, but there are still other techniques we can add.

Information

The client is blowing too hard, and it is distorting the sound production. The clinician adds behavior information about the sound production. She says to the client, "When you are making the sound, don't blow the air out so hard. Blow the air out gently. Listen to me again—[s]." With information added to the model and guidance, the client again improves his sound production and is rewarded.

Reward/Token Economy

We began with shaping behavior through rewards for behaviors that more closely approximated the correct behavior. We then added modeling, guidance, and information. Now, let us examine more carefully the reward itself and the procedure used to present the reward.

As the client is making attempts to produce the [s] sound, some of the attempts will more closely approximate the correct production than others. After each of these attempts, the clinician rewards him. She has decided that she will present a primary reward, a jelly bean, for each good production. If the client likes jelly beans, he will be motivated to produce the correct sound. This will increase the occurrence of the correct production. The clinician might be able to create even greater approach motivation if she rewards him with two jelly beans.

If the clinician has decided to use a token economy, she would give the client a token after each satisfactory production of the sound. She has some checkers in her desk that she uses as tokens. She first explains to the client that he will be able to buy some things from her "store" after therapy. She then shows him the items she has for rewards. She might have, for example, some candy or small toys, each with a token price on it. After explaining this, she initiates therapy, giving a token for good responses. After the therapy session is completed, she opens the store and allows the client to purchase anything he can afford. It is very important that the clinician have some items priced very low so the client can always purchase some reward from the store. A reward of two tokens might provide more approach motivation. The strength of the rewards is indeed important.

Penalty Not errorless learning

We have now dealt with rewarding good productions of the sound. How are we going to respond to those attempts the client makes that are not satisfactory? We have already discussed the disadvantages of trying to extinguish the behavior by not responding. Let us add another dimension to our therapy. Like a farmer trying to get a mule to move, we will not only dangle a carrot—the reward (R+)—in front of him, we will also be behind him with a big stick—punishment (P)—in case he stops. To mix metaphors, our clinical vehicle now has both front and rear wheel drive.

The clinician has been giving the client jelly beans for each good production of the [s] sound. She has the client save the jelly beans to eat after therapy, so as not to interfere with the clinical process. They are in a small cup in front of the client. She now tells him that every time he makes the sound incorrectly, she is going to take back one jelly bean. If the jelly beans are really important to the client, he will make every effort possible not to lose any of them (just as you would do to avoid losing the $5 every time you were late to class or work). The clinician could increase the client's avoidance motivation by removing two jelly beans for each incorrect production. The strength of this penalty is directly related to how many jelly beans he receives for correct production. If he receives only one jelly bean, but loses two, there is an increase in avoidance motivation. Here we have another ratio that we can control. If the client loses only one jelly bean but gets two for correct production, we are focusing on approach motivation, but avoidance motivation is still a factor.

This same situation would exist if the clinician were using a token economy, where she removed a token for an incorrect production. She might increase the client's avoidance motivation if she removed two or even three tokens for an incorrect response. Our therapy now is doubly efficient. We are not only encouraging the correct responses through rewards, we are discouraging the incorrect responses through penalty. There are many variations the clinician can use in terms of the ratio or amount of reward and penalty in the token economy. If approach motivation is the key, the reward consists of two tokens while the penalty remains at one token. If the clinician wants to focus on avoidance motivation, the penalty could be two tokens and the reward one token. Approach motivation and avoidance motivation are different factors in therapy, and the clinician may find herself using approach motivation during one phase of treatment and avoidance motivation in another.

When we are using rewards for the correct behavior and penalty for the incorrect behavior, our therapy is very efficient. Not only is the client trying to avoid the penalty by not producing the incorrect behavior, he is producing the correct behavior in order to get the reward. With this system, the correct behavior is being rewarded twice. The first reward is for the occurrence of the behavior while the second reward, a negative reward, is for the successful avoidance of the penalty. This is a very strong reward system. It is much stronger than only rewarding the correct productions and ignoring the incorrect productions. And when I say ignore the incorrect productions, I mean just that. If a clinician is drilling a particular sound with a client and is presenting a token reward for each correct production and making no response to the incorrect productions, she is using a reward-oriented token economy. But if she is giving tokens for correct productions and withholding tokens for incorrect productions, as well as telling the client that the production was wrong, she is using both rewards and penalties.

Clinical Transactions: The CIM

Initiating the First Transaction

Clinician to Client. At this point in our therapy, we have evaluated the client and determined what the problem is. We have also decided on the behavior change goal and have established rapport with our client. We are now ready to start the clinical process and teach the new behavior to the client. The first interaction between us and the client is the initial stimulus–organism/cognition–response cycle (S–O–R), where we present the first stimulus to the client. We have three choices of a stimulus, as seen earlier in Figure 3.5 in Chapter 3. We can provide any combination of modeling the behavior, guidance in the production of the behavior, or information about the behavior. Our choice of stimulus depends on what we hope to accomplish during our therapy session with the client and on any limitations our client might have, such as lower cognitive functioning, a hearing problem, or visual problems.

If we are attempting to teach the client a behavior that can easily be seen and/or heard, we can use a model of the behavior. We may also want to include some information in this first contact with the client. Consider the following statement by a clinician: "We are going to learn to make the [s] sound today. It is a hissing sound, something like a snake makes. We hold our teeth close together, put the tongue up behind the teeth, and blow air out gently. Listen to me make the sound and then you try it—[s]." This clinician started the transaction by giving the client information about the sound and modeling it for him.

Another example might be the clinician working with an older client who stutters. The clinician has decided that she is going to work on the rate of speech. She could say, "Most people who stutter have a tendency to talk too fast. Research has shown that people who stutter do not have the same degree of fine motor skills as people who do not stutter. Speech is a fine motor skill, and when the person who stutters talks too fast, he is more likely to have the speech system break down. I am talking to you at the rate of speech I want you to imitate. Let me hear you count to 10 using this rate." Again, we have information and a model. This clinician might possibly decide to use a *delayed auditory feedback* (DAF) to get the client to slow down his rate. The DAF does not model slow speech for the stutterer, but it does guide him to slower speech. To introduce this into therapy, she could give the same information as before but then add, "This is a Delayed Auditory Feedback, a DAF. You will hear your own speech in the earphones I put on you, but your speech will sound slower than you think it is. It will sound like an echo. You will have to talk slower when you are on the DAF. Now, let's put on the earphones, and when I signal, you count to 10."

When we make our stimulus choice to use in this initial contact, we must also consider the cognitive level of the client. If we present a model or information beyond the cognitive level of the client, it is inappropriate. The client will not comprehend what we are trying to teach. How do we determine the cognitive skills of the client? We should have some insight into his cognitive level from our initial evaluation. This first presentation is based on what we have already learned about the client's cognitive level, but we may still present the stimuli at too complex a level. We will be adjusting our stimuli to the client's cognitive level during the first several transactions. This is part of the testing process that is included in each transaction.

Our testing of cognitive awareness and perception will be based on the resultant response of the client, the R in our diagram. If we present the [s] sound and the client produces a sound totally unrelated to the model, our test indicates that the model was probably inappropriate. Either the model was too complex or the client did not receive enough information from the model to reproduce it. It could also be that the client is responding too fast, not giving himself time to process the information he received from the model. We can slow down the response by telling him not to respond until we give him a signal of some sort.

If we then add information to the model and the same response occurs, the test again indicates that the stimulus we provided was not appropriate. We must continue to modify the stimulus until the client can comprehend it. The client's degree of comprehension is the core of the second half of the initial transaction.

Client to Clinician. The response of the client is the stimulus for the clinician in the second half of our transaction. The model we are working on now is S–O–R/S–O–R. This is the testing and decision making part of the transaction. The clinician perceived the client's response and evaluated it first in terms of correctness, completeness, and frequency of occurrence. If the response indicated that the client comprehended the initial stimulus and was able to produce an improved response, the clinician has established an appropriate level of stimulus for the client.

The clinician must then decide how she will respond to the client and what form of reward she will present. Of course, the reward should have been determined before the therapy began, but some clinicians prefer to give spontaneous rewards. This preference is often the result of forgetting to plan therapy, and the rewards usually take the form of verbal praise such as "Very good, Johnny!" The major problem with this type of reward is its repetition; it all becomes meaningless. Some clinicians use an abbreviated form of praise, simply saying "Good." This is even more meaningless. This form of praise even becomes meaningless to the clinician because she simply mouths the words. If the clinician were to observe the effect this reward has on the speech of the client, she would realize that it is not effective. It would be much more effective if the clinician combined her verbal praise with a token. The reward is very important for the approach motivation of the client, and the approach motivation is very important to the success of therapy; if the client is not interested in coming for therapy, we are going to have clinical problems. One of the best rewards we can give a client is fun therapy. Therapy does not have to be tedious to be effective; if it is tedious, it is because the clinician views therapy that way.

If the client's response was not satisfactory, the clinician must reevaluate her stimuli and also respond in some way. Because this is the first transaction, the penalty, if given, should be carefully adjusted in terms of its strength. In other words, be gentle. The clinician might possibly respond by saying, "You made a good try." This rewards the effort the client made but also tells him that the response was not satisfactory. For most clients, this is too early in therapy to focus on the avoidance motivation of the client; in the early part of therapy, our approach should be as positive as possible. Nevertheless, we will encounter situations in which we have to focus on avoidance motivation early in therapy. This is especially true for those clients for whom we are unable to find an appropriate reward. These clients are few and far between, but they do exist.

Since we are still in the first clinical transaction, the effect of the reward or the penalty has not had an opportunity to influence either the frequency of occurrence of the speech behavior or the attending behaviors of the client. We need to sit down and think through our clinical approach very carefully if we have lost the client this early in therapy! We will begin monitoring the influences of the reward and penalty after therapy has progressed a bit further.

Before concluding the first transaction, the clinician must decide what her next stimulus will be to initiate the second transaction. If the initial stimulus did not achieve the desired results and the client's response was not satisfactory, the next stimulus must be modified. The model must be made slower and clearer. More information could be provided to clarify the behavior for the client. The clinician might even decide to add guidance to the stimulus. It is possible to combine all three stimuli in introducing the next transaction. It would be feasible for the clinician to combine them by saying, "When you just made the [s] sound, your lower lip was too high and the sound could not get out. When you make it this time, I am going to hold your lower lip down so the sound can get out. Now, listen and watch me make the sound and then you try it again—[s]." She then holds the client's lower lip down while he makes the next attempt. She has used modeling, guidance, and information. If she must modify this stimulus even more in the future, she can expand the amount of information by explaining the sound production more carefully, exaggerating the production of the model of the sound, and exerting even more guidance on the lower lip.

When the client's response is satisfactory at this step of shaping, the clinician then moves ahead in therapy. She provides a stimulus that moves the behavioral production to the next step in successive approximation.

Initiating the Second Transaction

As you can see in the CIM, the clinician has determined the stimulus and the direction of the next transaction before the first transaction is completed. She then terminates the first transaction with her response and starts the next one with her stimulus. For example, the clinician might say, "That was a pretty good sound, David, but I think you can do it better" (response-penalty). "Now, watch me again. I will do it slower this time so you can see exactly how I do it. Watch how I hold my teeth together—[ssss]" (stimulus, information, and model). The second transaction is now underway with the client perceiving the stimulus, thinking about it, and then responding. If the client's response is too fast, it can be slowed down by introducing a signal for the client to respond. (Remember, the efficiency of therapy is not dependent on the speed of the client's response.) The clinician again evaluates the response, decides how she will respond, and determines her stimulus to initiate the next transaction. The transactions now continue with the clinician and the client playing their respective roles.

As the transactions continue, the clinician becomes more involved in monitoring the second transactional mode, which includes the effects of the reward and penalty both on the frequency of occurrence of speech behaviors and on the client's approach motivation and/or avoidance motivation. These factors become more influential as the client gains extended experience with the reward and penalty system. He must develop approach motivation to get the reward and avoidance motivation to avoid the penalty. This is part of the cognitive function of the client in therapy.

Ongoing Transactions

Therapy is now underway. Each transaction builds on the preceding one. The clinician uses shaping—steps of successive approximation—to bring the behavior closer and closer to the behavior change goal. She continues to model and give information and guidance as the behavior changes. The better productions of the behavior are rewarded while the poorer productions are penalized. She is using a constant reward schedule because it results in quicker learning. As the behavior begins to stabilize, she fades the model, information, and guidance until the behavior occurs without assistance. She continues to monitor the second transactional mode, keeping track of the client's attentiveness and frequency of occurrence of the speech behaviors. She may have to adjust her reward and/or penalty, but this can be done quickly so that therapy can proceed. We complete this step in the clinical process when the behavior occurs spontaneously or through a gestural prompt. We are still rewarding each occurrence, but there is no penalty since the behavior is stable and production errors no longer occur.

Keep in mind that we have two basic modes of clinical transaction: one focused on *speech* behavior and the other on *attending* behavior. If the client is attending to therapy and the speech behavior is responding appropriately to either reward or penalty, the attending behavior is only monitored. However, if a problem arises in terms of the client's attending to therapy, the transactions shift to the secondary mode where the focus is on the attending behavior. We can improve the client's attending to therapy either through his approach motivation or his avoidance motivation.

Stimulus Manipulation

Role Shift

In this early stage of treatment, we are not going to be concerned with all three categories of stimuli (people, talking situations, and objects). We are going to concentrate on shifting stimulus roles of the various people in our client's nonclinical environments. Obviously there are going to be many instances in therapy where we will not have an opportunity to work either directly or indirectly with significant others in our client's lives. This shortcoming is going to have an adverse effect on our therapy because the client will not have a "support system" as he goes through therapy.

If we are able to work with the significant others, it might be worthwhile to consider their stimulus roles before we come in contact with the client. Regardless of the type of communication disorder, the significant others are either rewarding the communication disorder or penalizing it. They either have a positive or negative reaction to the disorder. In either event, it would be wise to minimize this influence before treatment begins. It would be problematic to penalize an incorrect behavior in the clinical environment while it was being rewarded in the home. At this point (as shown in Figure 7.1), the significant others' role is shifted to that of an SO. There is no way we can completely eliminate all positive or negative reactions made by the signifi-

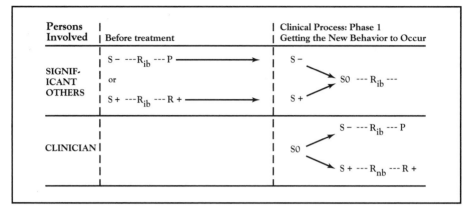

Figure 7.1. Stimulus role shift model—Clinical process: Phase 1. Before treatment, the significant others either directly or indirectly reward or penalize the incorrect behavior. Their stimulus roles are then either an $S+$ (reward) or an $S-$ (penalty). The clinician is not yet involved with the client or the significant others. As treatment starts Phase 1, the influence of the significant others is neutralized by shifting their stimulus' roles from an $S+$ or an $S-$ to an $S0$, neither rewarding nor penalizing the incorrect behavior. The clinician shifts her stimulus role from a neutral stimulus, $S0$, to an $S+$, rewarding the new behavior, and an $S-$, penalizing the incorrect behavior.

cant others, but we can reduce them and their effects through counseling the signifigant others and instructing them to respond in a more neutral manner. In the same vein the clinician shifts from her $S0$ role before therapy to an $S+$ for the new behavior and an $S-$ for the old behavior as therapy begins. Her role shift is accomplished through her association with the rewards and penalties.

Gradual Introduction of Stimuli

The gradual introduction of stimuli has little value at this stage of therapy. It would only apply to such things as a gradual increase in the amount of information we might use as part of the stimulus, or a gradual increase in the amount of physical guidance we provide a client. This form of manipulation will be important in later stages of therapy.

Gradual Withdrawal of Stimuli

Gradual withdrawal of stimuli is an important function in that we must gradually withdraw or fade the stimuli used to create the new behavior. As the behavior becomes more stable, we can fade the model, the information, and the guidance. We can fade all three at the same time, or we can fade one at a time. Fading may involve decreasing the frequency of occurrence of guidance, the intensity or strength of a model, the duration or completeness of information, or any combination of these with any stimuli.

Increase the Number of Stimuli

This stimulus manipulation method is not extremely important in this therapy phase. The only way we use it is by adding guidance and then information to the model. We increase the number of stimuli that make up the stimulus to initiate each clinical transaction.

Decreasing the Number of Stimuli

At this early stage of therapy, we are limited to decreasing the number of S+ and S− that are associated with the communication disorder. This is limited to shifting the roles of the significant others in the client's most immediate environment.

Clinical Examples

Now that we have covered all the pertinent information regarding the CIM model, let us take time to consider several clinical examples. We will take several clients and adjust the CIM model to the particular client by manipulating the antecedent events. We will then consider other clients with whom we will have to manipulate contingent events to the unique needs of the client. If you see some factors that should have been considered and I overlooked, remember that "To err is human, to forgive divine."

Manipulating the Antecedent Events

Example 1. Our client is an 8-year-old girl with a high-frequency hearing loss and a resultant distortion of the sibilants. It is our decision to begin work on the [s] sound. We normally model the sound for the client and see if the client can imitate the sound. However, we recognize that the high-frequency hearing loss may prevent the client from perceiving the model correctly. This does not mean that we cannot use the auditory channel. We can still use it for behavioral information. We can use the model of the sound, but it will be aimed primarily at the visual channel so the client can see the articulatory position to assume for the correct production. We then supplement the model with behavioral information concerning the placement of the articulators. Information concerning the sound's quality is not appropriate here because of the hearing problem. The client really does not know how a snake sounds. If this stimulus is not sufficient to produce a better [s] sound, we can also introduce physical guidance for the articulatory position. In this instance, we might use a tongue blade to provide physical guidance of the lips and positioning of the teeth. Using your fingers is frowned on in most clinical settings; bites can be painful. With each presentation of the stimuli, we shape the production of the [s] sound. Although the client may not be able to hear the subtle changes we make in the [s] production, she will be able to discern the physical changes in the positioning of the articulators. In this particular instance, we modify our behavior change goal from a perfect [s] production to an acceptable one because there is an organic factor involved in the error. The physical monitoring of the production by the client is not as accurate and reliable as auditory monitoring would be. We now have adjusted our stimuli to the limitations of the client, using as much of the auditory channel as is practical and supplementing it with the visual and body sense channels.

Example 2. This client is a 7-year-old boy who omits the [ɝ] sound. One of the problems in teaching this sound is that the unique tongue position for the sound is not visible. If you open your mouth wide during the production of the sound so that the client can see it, the tongue position and the sound itself are distorted. Thus, the model is somewhat limited in terms of visual information concerning the placement of the tongue. In order to expand the stimuli, we add behavioral information, telling the client where to put his tongue and how to hold it. Again, we might provide physical guidance with a tongue blade to help the client get the tongue where it should be. Another type of guidance might be verbal guidance, where we tell the client to make the sound of a fire engine. The client might be able to produce the [ɝ] sound in this context, but not when asked to produce the sound as a phoneme. If the fire engine fails, try a police car.

Example 3. This client is a man with expressive aphasia and severe apraxia. He cannot voluntarily control any of his articulators. He cannot even open his mouth upon command. For all intents and purposes, the client is nonverbal, although he makes grunting sounds that appear to have no significance. Our evaluation indicates that he comprehends at a relatively normal level. The first tasks we set for ourselves are to increase voluntary control over the articulators and to start opening the mouth. We model the behavior, and the client struggles but cannot perform the behavior. We then verbally request the client to open his mouth as we model the behavior. Again, the client attempts to follow the instructions but is unable to do so. Because this is an apraxia, we know that behaviors can occur on a reflex level even though they cannot be performed voluntarily. What can we use to elicit a reflexive opening of the mouth? The most obvious stimulus would seem to be a spoon. Turning to environmental guidance, we take the spoon and place it at the client's mouth. The client's mouth opens reflexively to receive food. We now have the behavior occurring, but we need to change the stimulus that cues the behavior from the spoon to the verbal request. We then pair the verbal request with the presentation of the spoon, saying, "Open your mouth" as the spoon is moved toward the mouth. We now begin to gradually withdraw the presentation of the spoon (fading this stimulus) as we continue to make the verbal request. After the association is made between the verbal request and the mouth opening, the response will occur without the spoon being present. In this instance, we bypassed the purely cognitive approach and start from a reflex level in order to get the behavior to occur.

Example 4. Let us consider another adult client. There is no apraxia with this woman, but there is a severe expressive aphasia. She has some expressive language but has difficulty naming objects. This is a transient problem, since many times she can recall the names of objects. This tells us that simply modeling the name of an object is useless since she already knows the name and how to say it. She just cannot recall the name at various times. We need to develop another cue that will assist the client in remembering the name when her normal recall procedures fail her. We decide that the word we want to work on is "cup." We bring a cup into therapy with us and, as we model the word for her to repeat, we have her look at the cup and pick it up as if to drink some coffee. We are now building associations between the word and the visual and motor cues. We can then gradually withdraw the model and introduce verbal guidance in the form of a question, such as "What do you drink coffee from?" We must be careful how we phrase the question. If we asked, "How do you drink your coffee?" the client might respond, "With cream and sugar." If the natural recall process fails here as she attempts to answer the question, she is able to look at the cup for additional cuing information. If this fails to cue the word, she can then pick up the cup as if to drink some coffee. She is adding still another cuing system to aid her recall of the word. We now have taught her to add visual and body sense cues to supplement the natural word recall process.

Example 5. This client is an 18-year-old woman who stutters. Our clinical goal is to reduce her speaking rate in order to achieve fluency. First of all, we try modeling the rate of speech we want, along with some behavioral information about how to speak slower. We find that even with the model, information, and verbal guidance in the form of cues or hints about the speech rate, the client is unable to slow her speech rate. We then put the client on a Delayed Auditory Feedback (DAF), where she hears her speech through earphones only after a .25-second delay. After some initial faltering, she begins to speak at a very slow rate. This is environmental guidance. We have manipulated her auditory environment in such a way that a slow speech rate is elicited. The DAF forces the slower rate of speech. We must now slowly remove the DAF as the behavior is maintained. We can do this by gradually reducing the amount of delay in the speech playback. This is a unique form of environmental guidance in that it is a clinical instrument that elicits or forces a response of slow speech. In this instance, we are changing the input signal in such a way that the speech rate is reduced. It is the DAF output, the delayed feedback, that provides the changed speech signal that produces the change in rate. In this way, the DAF is a stimulus, an environmental guidance stimulus.

Manipulating the Contingent Events

Example 1. Our client in this example is a 5-year-old boy with a slight articulation disorder. When the client first came in for therapy, he paid close attention to the therapy and seemed to enjoy his time with us. He made good progress on his speech and was rewarded with colored stars that were stuck on his work papers. However, as the novelty of the clinical experience wore off, the child gradually began to lose interest in therapy. He would daydream during therapy, and clinical progress was flagging. We were aware of both types of clinical transactions, speech behavior and attending behavior, and, although we had been focusing on the speech behavior transactions, we were monitoring the attending behaviors. As the client's attending behaviors began to fade, we recognized that the efficiency of our therapy was also fading. We could not teach him if he was not paying attention. In order to correct this situation we shifted our clinical focus to the attending behavior transactions. The first thing we have to recognize is that our reward is no longer actually rewarding to the client. He has received so many stars that they no longer have value to him. So we either have to change our reward in order to achieve approach motivation or introduce a penalty to achieve avoidance motivation. Either approach motivation and avoidance motivation will get the attending behavior for us. How do we decide which will be more effective? Let us first consider that things went very well in therapy until the reward lost its value. The easiest thing to do would be to find another form of reward. We are working with eight other children in this agency, and several of them have also tired of their rewards. So we decide to use a token economy on all of our clients. We gather a number of what we hope are interesting items that could serve as rewards. We have trinkets, gum, candy, and various small toys. We keep these "goodies" in a container. This, then, constitutes our store. The first day we change over to the token economy, we make sure that each client gets some tokens, and then we open our store. When they make their first purchases, the association is made between the tokens and the backup rewards. Now they are hooked. There are so many things to choose from. They like several things, but they can only afford one item each time the store is open. Then there is inflation. Clinicians soon learn to set the prices high enough so that they are not spending half their salary on rewards. With this reward system, we have greatly reduced the chances of our client losing interest in his rewards. A wide variety of rewards is available, and he gets his choice of the one that is most important to him.

We now shift our clinical focus to attending behaviors, and when the client is attending, we give him a token. The token might be given to him for a correct response to a model, but the correct response indicates that he was attending. With his increased interest in achieving the reward, we now have approach motivation to perform the behaviors that will be rewarded. Once we have regained the client's attending behavior and approach motivation, we can shift back to the speech behavior transactions, although we will continue to monitor the client's attending behavior.

Example 2. We are now faced with a 16-year-old girl who has severe language delay—possibly a working vocabulary of 35 words, 20 of which cannot be printed in this book. Her comprehension is good, even though the records indicate rather extensive brain injury at birth. The client is emotionally impaired and demonstrates aggressive behavior toward teachers and therapists. On the first day of therapy, we took her into the clinic room and started our first clinical transaction. Her response was to spit on us. Each time we presented her with a stimulus, her response was to spit. Should we try to extinguish the behavior by ignoring it? How do you ignore someone who is spitting on you? Obviously we cannot start therapy until we deal with this behavior. We must deal directly with this behavior by finding a contingent event that influences the frequency of occurrence of the spitting. Our client finds the behavior itself rewarding so we must find a penalty that is stronger than the reward she is experiencing. The first thing we try is spitting back at her (crude, perhaps, but practical). She enjoys this (it is a reward), and her spitting increases in frequency. We then decide that when she spits we will hold her hands firmly in her lap for one minute. When we do this, the client becomes quite agitated. We carefully explain that if she spits on us we will hold her hands in her lap for a period of time. We now find that the occurrence of spitting behavior lessens. The client is developing avoidance motivation toward the unpleasant experience of having her hands held in her lap. Our clinical role with the client is changing. She has associated us with the penalty for spitting. We have become an S− for the spitting behavior. When she sees us, she is cued that if the spitting occurs she will be penalized. So in our presence, there is no longer any spitting behavior. However, the spitting behavior will continue to occur at the same level in other environments, where there is no S− to cue the penalty. We can now move on to basic treatment procedures with this client.

Example 3. We are now going to deal with a 35-year-old man who stutters. Our clinical goal is to establish a slower rate of speech. He is able to follow the model of rate we are providing. We are going to start shaping his speech rate by rewarding his speech when it approximates the speech rate we want. In our conversations with the client, we are careful to model the desired rate of speech. When he answers us, we will determine if his speech rate is closer to our model and, if so, he is rewarded. However, there are many instances where his speech rate is much too fast. In order to make our therapy more efficient, we decide that we are not going to ignore these fast speech episodes, we are going to penalize them. Our main problem now is to create appropriate rewards and penalties for an adult. If the way to a man's heart is through his stomach, the way to his approach motivation and avoidance motivation is through his wallet. We have the client bring in $2 in dimes, and we set up the contingencies. Each time he produces a slower rate of speech that approximates our model, he gets 20¢ back. Every time he speaks too fast, he loses 10¢. The client now has a great deal of approach motivation to get back his $2 by performing at the correct rate. He also has the avoidance motivation to avoid losing his money by speaking too fast. What does he substitute for his fast talking? Slow talking. The slow talking then is directly rewarded by his receiving 20¢ and negatively rewarded by his not losing 10¢. This particular arrangement is biased toward the reward side of the economy. Then, later in therapy, our client becomes a bit lazy. He can receive four rewards, and this will cancel out eight penalties (a little exercise in higher math). We want to stress the elimination of the fast rate of speech, so we change the economy so that each episode of slow talking is rewarded by 10¢ but each instance of fast talking is penalized by the loss of 30¢. We have now reversed the focal point of the economy. We are now concentrating on the penalty, providing the client with much avoidance motivation to avoid losing his money. The approach motivation is still operating (10¢ worth), but the prime mover is the avoidance motivation to avoid losing 30¢ each time the rate is too fast.

As this is all transpiring, we are assuming new roles in the clinic room. When we are rewarding proper rate, we assume the role of S, cuing this behavior to occur. As we penalize the fast rate we become an S−, cuing the faster speech not to occur. In order to maintain these roles we must continue to reward and penalize. This creates no problem, since we are in the phase of therapy where we are using constant reward when the correct behavior occurs and constant penalty when the fast rate occurs.

Planning and Problem Solving

The following clinical situations are for you to ponder. Each will pose a problem in either planning an appropriate stimulus, selecting an appropriate reward/penalty system, or solving a problem encountered in an ongoing clinical interaction. Review each situation carefully and then write down your analysis of the situation and what you would do. After you have finished all of the clinical situations, turn to Appendix D, where each situation is discussed. These discussions are not meant to be the answers, but rather a discussion of important points to consider and possible solutions. There are no single solutions to these situations.

Situation A

The evaluation of this 17-year-old boy indicates that he is rather severely retarded in terms of language skills. Even his limited vocabulary is difficult to understand because of poor motor control over the articulatory system. The history indicates brain injury at birth and general mental retardation. An audiological report states that the client could not be adequately tested, but there appears to be a rather significant hearing loss in both ears. The client is in a foster care facility where he must be able to let his needs and wants be known. The problem is that he has neither the vocabulary nor the articulatory skills to communicate his needs. Your task is to create a clinical program to teach this client a basic needs vocabulary that other people can understand. You should concentrate your planning on an appropriate stimulus system for this client.

Situation B

Your client is a 45-year-old man who has recently had a laryngectomy. He is discouraged about ever learning to talk again. You have this client in individual therapy 3 days a week. Your task is to teach him to use esophageal speech. Your primary focus should be on the types of stimuli you are going to use with this client. Also, discuss the ways you might use contingent events with this client.

Situation C

This client is a 7-year-old girl with an articulation disorder. There is nothing significant about the girl's case except that she comes from a wealthy family who has doted on her every whim. In nontechnical language, she is spoiled rotten. If there is something she does not have, it is only because she does not want it. You must plan your contingencies around this.

Situation D

This 9-year-old boy has a rather severe voice disorder. He has had an examination by a physician, who reported that he has vocal nodes. Your evaluation indicates that a good share of the vocal abuse was due to his use of sudden vocal onset (hard vocal attack or onset) as part of his speech. How would you teach new vocal behavior to the client? How would you introduce other factors involved in vocal abuse?

C H A P T E R

8

HABITUATING THE NEW BEHAVIOR

◆ Synopsis

We have now progressed to the point where the new behavior is occurring consistently in the clinical environment, although it is still dependent on prompts or cues and the reward. We now need to stabilize it and make it independent of prompts, cues, and rewards. The behavior must be habituated in the clinical environment before we can generalize it to other environments. We must gradually wean the behavior from the prompts, cues, and rewards and then test it to see if it is stable and habituated. This chapter will discuss how this is achieved in this phase of therapy via the Clinical Interaction Model (CIM).

Antecedent and Contingent Events in the CIM

At this phase of the clinical process, the new behavior is stable in the clinic room, but it is still somewhat dependent on prompts or cues and the reward. We have continued with a constant reward program up to this point in therapy. If you get the feeling this step overlaps with the last step, you are right. It is very hard to differentiate between the last stages of getting the behavior to occur and the first stages of habituating the behavior. There is no clear line of demarcation, no clear-cut border. We will be using different strategies in this step, so we will discuss it as a separate phase of therapy. Our task here is to make the behavior independent of the prompts, cues, and rewards.

The focus in this phase of therapy is on the contingent events. The reward schedule we have used up to this point was designed for quick learning. But when a constant schedule of reward is removed, the behavior quickly extinguishes. In this phase of the clinical process, we must change the schedule to intermittent rewards. With this schedule, behaviors become very stable and quite independent of the reward. It is almost impossible to extinguish a behavior that has been learned on an intermittent reward schedule. When we use this reward schedule, our client never knows when he is going to receive a reward. He may perform the behavior three times with no reward and then on the fourth time he gets the reward. He continues to perform the behavior, waiting for the reward. This practice of the behavior without the reward is the important part of habituation. Many people in our society have been trained to gamble as a result of this type of reward schedule. Consider the slot machine. You put in five coins with no reward and then with the sixth coin you receive four coins back. Unless your math is extremely poor, you recognize that you are still two coins short. But do you stop? No, you are encouraged to play more coins in the hope that you will receive another reward, maybe even the jackpot. So you put back the four coins you received plus five more before you are rewarded again. This time you are paid off with 15 coins and you are 6 coins ahead. This is obviously the time to stop playing. However, there is that human element called greed, and this keeps most people playing. You do not stop and think about your chances of winning, you only know that there is a chance that you will win big. Of course, in this example we have two factors operating, intermittent reward and greed. If you have ever been to a gambling casino, you have probably noticed people who sit between two slot machines and play them both for hours on end, perhaps even days on end. They are hooked. Intermittent reward is a powerful learning tool.

Fading Antecedent Events

In the previous phase of therapy, we had a series of antecedent events that we used to get the new behavior to occur. We faded or withdrew most of these events toward the end of that phase of therapy. The model was no longer needed. But we did continue to use environmental, verbal, and gestural guidance to prompt the new behavior. We did things like show the client pictures that would prompt the behavior, verbally request the behavior, or gesture in such a way that the client would perform the behavior. The behavior did not yet occur spontaneously.

Now we want to withdraw these cues so the behavior occurs spontaneously. For example, instead of using pictures that are aimed directly at prompting the behavior, such as a picture of a snake for the [s] sound or a cup to prompt the word, we would use more subtle cues. We might use a general picture with many objects, and see if the [s] sound occurs, or we could use a saucer and see if the word "cup" is produced. This process would be applied to verbal and gestural cues. The cues are modified to more subtle forms and once the behavior is occurring with these subtle prompts, we can remove the prompts and the behavior will occur spontaneously. The withdrawal process must be gradual, allowing the client to adjust to more subtle cues.

Fading the Contingent Events

Let us first consider the role of penalty in the habituation of the new behavior. Penalty plays a minor role if it plays any role at all. We have established the behavior in the previous step of therapy, and the error is no longer occurring. Therefore, we no longer need to penalize incorrect productions. However, in some clinical instances, we might have to incorporate penalty to a minor degree. If we are working with a client who has an articulation problem and we are incorporating the new sound into words, we may have to back up a bit in the clinical process to get the new sound to occur in specific words as we are habituating. In this instance we would use penalty. So let us not totally abandon the concept of penalty in this step of therapy. As the error occurs less often, though, the penalty will be faded.

The gradual withdrawal of the reward is extremely important. In the previous phase of therapy, we were rewarding each and every performance of the behavior. Now, if we suddenly take away the reward, the behavior will extinguish; it will gradually disappear. We must change the schedule of presentation of the reward. We have choices regarding how to switch to an intermittent reward schedule. We can base our presentation of the reward on either the number of times the behavior is performed before it is rewarded (ratio system) or we can use time as a factor (interval system).

There are two types of ratio systems: fixed and variable. If we decide on a fixed ratio system, we decide that the client will receive a reward after an exact number of performances. If we have a ratio of 3:1, this means that he receives the reward on every fourth performance. With a variable ratio system, we do not stick to a constant number of performances before giving the reward. The client might perform the behavior two times and receive a reward and then perform it five times before the next reward. The system is constantly varying according to the clinician's choices.

With the interval (i.e., time-based) reward schedule, we again have two choices: the fixed interval and the variable interval. The fixed interval means that we reward the client after a standard period of time, while the variable interval calls for rewards to be presented according to variable intervals of time.

In my clinical experience, I have found that the interval system is not practical for most speech behaviors. What do you do if, within the time interval you have selected, the client does not perform the behavior? This type of schedule does not appear to fit the general needs of the speech clinician. However, if you are attempting to increase the duration of a behavior, such as paying attention or sitting in a chair, the interval system is ideal.

The fixed and variable interval systems of reward presentation have a unique application for the speech clinician, but we will be using the fixed and variable ratio schedules in most of our therapy. I have used them and found that they both work very well in therapy. My main problem with the fixed ratio was that I had to keep counting the number of times the client performed the behavior so that I could reward him appropriately. Because counting distracts my attention from therapy, I shifted to the variable ratio and found that I was very comfortable with it.

With either ratio schedule, however, it is important that the reward occur less and less often as habituation occurs. With the fixed ratio schedule, the ratio would have to increase over time. The clinician might start with a 3:1 ratio but then shift to 4:1, 5:1, and so on. With the variable ratio schedule, the clinician would have to make sure that the number of performances increases before the reward is given. Eventually, say when the client receives a reward after 20 performances, the behavior is not dependent on the reward, and the reward can be completely removed.

Testing Habituation

If the reward is removed and the behavior continues to occur, it is habituated. You might view this as an indication that the behavior itself has become rewarding. In any event, after the reward has been removed and the behavior continues to occur, the behavior has been habituated and will occur spontaneously with no prompts and no reward from the clinician. But what are we going to do if, when we remove the reward, the behavior begins to falter? We must go back to our reward schedule at a level where the behavior is occurring again. Once we have the behavior stable at this level, we reinstate the withdrawal program. What does all this tell us? It tells us that we moved too quickly in the removal of the reward. If patience is a virtue, then all speech clinicians must be virtuous.

Stimulus Manipulation

Role Shift

As we move into the second phase of the clinical process, we are still going to concentrate on the people in the client's environment. We also begin to consider the other types of stimuli, talking situations, and objects. Let us consider each of these in order.

Significant Others and the Clinician. It is now time to shift the significant other's role from that of an S0 (established while the new behavior was being created) to that of an S+ for the new behavior and an S for the old behavior. This is done so that the generalization process can begin. It is accomplished by having the significant others begin to reward the new behavior when it occurs in the external environment and to penalize the old behavior when it occurs (see Figure 8.1).

This process of shifting roles should not be done immediately, but should occur while the client is still in this phase of the clinical process. The clinician must carefully identify for the significant others what the new behavior is, determine what the reward will be, and decide how often the reward is presented.

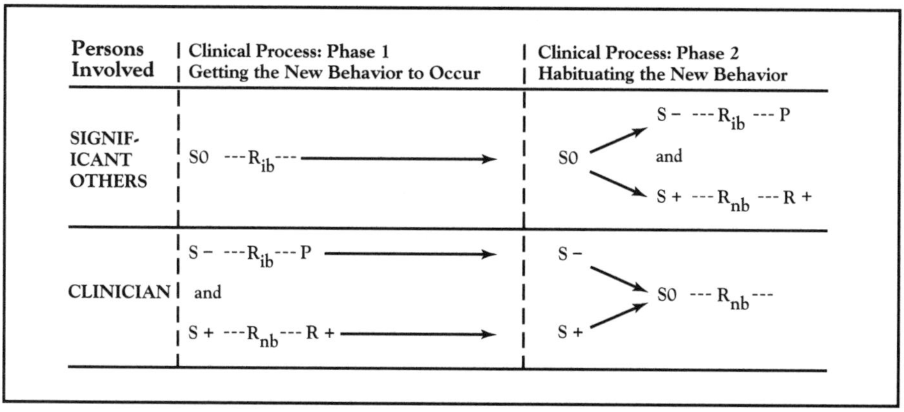

Persons Involved	Clinical Process: Phase 1 Getting the New Behavior to Occur	Clinical Process: Phase 2 Habituating the New Behavior
SIGNIFICANT OTHERS	S0 ---R_{ib}--- ⟶	S0 ⟨ S− ---R_{ib}--- P and S+ ---R_{nb}--- R +
CLINICIAN	S− ---R_{ib}--- P ⟶ and S+ ---R_{nb}--- R + ⟶	S− ⟩ S0 ---R_{nb}--- S+

Figure 8.1. Stimulus role shift model—Clinical process: Phase 2. As treatment progresses from Phase 1 to Phase 2, the significant others' stimulus roles are shifted from that of an S0 to an S+, rewarding the new behavior, and an S−, penalizing the incorrect behavior in order to encourage the new behavior to begin to occur in the external environment. To test the habituation of the new behavior in the clinical environment, the clinician shifts her stimulus roles from S+ and S− to that of an S0. In doing this, she removes the contingent rewards to test the stability of the new behavior.

If a token system is employed, the type of token reward and the backup rewards must be determined. It is also important that the significant others start with a constant reward schedule, so that the new behavior is encouraged in the external environment.

As the roles of the significant others are shifting, the clinician is also shifting her roles. In the previous step, she had been an S+ for the new behavior and an S− for the old behavior. The old behavior was occurring less and less, so the need for penalty diminished. As this occurred, the clinician's role of S− faded, but the role of S+ was even stronger, because she was rewarding all occurrences and, by the end of this step, all occurrences were correct. She now begins to withdraw the reward by changing the schedule of reward from a constant schedule to an intermittent schedule. When the new behavior occurs and the clinician does not reward it, she begins to assume the role of S0. The role of S0 becomes more and more important as the ratio of reward changes. When the ratio is 1:1, she is an S0 half of the time, but when the ratio is 5:1, the role of S0 occurs 80% of the time. In this way the clinician slowly assumes the role of S0, testing the habituation of the new behavior in the clinical environment.

Other Stimuli. In many instances it will be very important for us to begin shifting the roles of other stimuli, talking situations, and objects while the therapy is still taking place in the clinical environment. This does not apply to all clients, only those where the S− are so strong that the client will need direct assistance in dealing with them. The factor that determines whether or not we will start role shifting in this phase of therapy seems to be the emotional involvement of the client with both his disorder and the stimuli. We will want to begin the role shift in the clinical environment, because we will have maximum control over the stimuli. Once the client is working alone in the external environment, our control over the stimuli is greatly reduced, and the client may not be able to perform the new speech behavior when confronted with the stimuli. Within the clinical environment, we can manipulate the stimuli in ways to encourage the new speech behavior to occur. We might view this early role shifting as a "halfway house" for the client. He is being provided with a means to deal with the S− situations in a controlled environment. This experience will increase the probability that he will be able to deal with the S− situations in the external environment.

Talking Situations. It might be important to start working on role shifts for talking situations while still in this step of the clinical process. This would be particularly appropriate for those clients who stutter. If a certain situation is an S− for the client, it could be dealt with initially in the clinical environment, where the clinician has control over the strength or intensity of the situation. She could begin to change the role of this situation through gradual introduction of the stimulus. This would include such talking situations as speaking before groups or talking to clerks in stores. The gradual introduction of the stimuli could be accomplished through techniques such as role playing and sociodramas (or whatever name the clinician uses to describe the process of creating situations in the clinic room that give the client an opportunity to practice his new speech behaviors in a controlled environment). Role shifting of talking situations in this step of therapy is usually reserved for special clients with special needs. It is not the rule; it is the exception.

Objects. As with talking situations, objects may need to be dealt with within the clinical environment. Objects that have the role of S− might include the telephone, dictating machines, tape recorders, public address systems, and other such communication devices. Object fear is usually associated with clients who stutter. It is often advisable to deal initially with these objects in the controlled clinical environment, as a form of prelude to generalizing the new behavior, the next step in our therapy. Gradual presentation of the stimulus object is used to begin to change the role of the object. With the telephone, the clinician might start with the easiest telephone situation and then gradually increase the difficulty. The first task of the client might be to look at a disconnected telephone while remaining calm. When the client can do this, he would touch the telephone, maintaining his composure. The next step would be to put the receiver to his ear. Subsequent steps would include dialing the telephone and asking for a specific person. This process can be used with other feared objects as well.

Gradual Introduction of Stimuli

It is evident from role shifting that this form of stimulus manipulation is used selectively in this step of therapy. Its use is limited to those S− stimuli that need to be dealt with in the clinical environment. This form of manipulation of talking situations and objects is not used with all types of clients.

As we are changing the roles of the significant others to S+ and S− as discussed above, we gradually introduce these new stimuli to the client. This is a gradual process, as the significant others become associated with rewards and penalties for specific behaviors. Also, as the clinician shifts her role from a strong S+ to an S0, her new role is gradually introduced.

Gradual Withdrawal of Stimuli

There is only limited use of this form of manipulation in this step of therapy. The clinician gradually withdraws rewards as the schedule of rewards changes. This results in the gradual withdrawal of the S+ role of the clinician. We also gradually withdraw the S0 role of the significant others as they assume their new roles of S+ and S−.

Increasing the Number of Stimuli

The stimuli we are dealing with here are the significant others. As we shift their roles, we are increasing the number of S+ for the new speech behavior and increasing the number of S− for the old behavior. Prior to this, the only S+ and S− the client associated with his speech were from the clinician. It is possible that the talking situations and objects that the clinician worked on in the clinical environment have also shifted their roles, and in this event, we would also be increasing the number of S+ to cue the new behavior. However, this role shift might still be limited to the clinic room, since the client has not dealt with the stimuli in the external environment.

Decreasing the Number of Stimuli

You have probably recognized by now that we are dealing with two types of S−. We are using one form of S− to discourage the occurrence of the old be-havior, and we are increasing the number of these stimuli. But we also have S− roles associated with specific talking situations and objects. These S− are indirectly associated with the incorrect speech behavior. They cue a negative emotional response in the client that interferes with the performance of the new speech behavior. We need to decrease the number of these S− in order for the client to be able to perform the new speech behavior in their presence. We accomplish this shift of the role of the stimuli through gradual introduc-tion of the stimuli in the clinical environment.

Clinical Examples

Fading the Antecedent Events

Example 1. Our client in this example is a 10-year-old boy who is nonverbal. We have taught him to say the word "water" in the previous step of therapy. The antecedent events we used were the model of the word and environmental guidance in the form of pictures of a lake and a glass of water. We used a to-ken economy as a reward system. We started out by giving him a drink of wa-ter after each production of the word, but we ran into two problems. First of all, he became satiated with water, and second, our therapy was constantly in-terrupted with his having to go to the bathroom. So we shifted to tokens, which he could use to purchase a drink of water when he wanted it. In the ha-bituation step of therapy, we would begin to fade the visual cues by using pic-tures that would include some aspect of water but not as a main theme. We might, for example, use a picture of a kitchen sink and a picture of a boat. We then gradually fade this type of cue, changing, perhaps, to taking the client to a sink and seeing if this environmental cue elicits the response.

Example 2. This client is a 15-year-old boy who stutters. We have established a slower rate of speech using the DAF. He is now speaking at the new rate while on the DAF, even though there is no delay in the speech signal he hears (we have faded the delay from .25 seconds to 0). In other words, he is hearing him-self normally through the DAF. We then begin to turn down the volume of the DAF so that eventually he can hear nothing through the earphones. The next step is to remove the earphones as he continues to talk at the new rate. We then move the DAF unit to another part of the clinic room. The final step is to remove the DAF from the clinic room.

Fading the Contingent Events

Because we are dealing with a single event in this section, we are limited to the number of clinical examples we can discuss since they would all be the same. We are concerned only with the frequency of presentation of the reward, regardless of whether we are using ratios or intervals. If we withdraw the re-ward too fast, the new behavior may begin to extinguish. We must then go back and provide rewards more often. Let us consider a single example and see if it can be generalized to all types of clients. In this example we are dealing with a 7-year-old girl who has been taught the [k] sound in words. The reward has been green stars, stuck in her speech book beside words she has been work-ing on. We now change to red stars so we can tell which stars have been given for which step in therapy. We use a variable ratio for the reward, being careful to give many stars as we start habituation. We then begin to fade the reward by not rewarding as often. During the second clinical session, we find that the production of the [k] in the words is slipping. We have moved too fast. So we back up and go to a heavier reward schedule. This will solve the problem. We are not faced with the problem that the client cannot make the sound in the word. We are dealing with the automaticity of the production. It has not been firmly established yet. When the client is attending carefully to the production, it is correct, but as the client attends to other things, the production slips. Back to the drawing board.

Role Shifting: Talking Situations and Objects

Example 1. Our client is a 55-year-old man who, as a result of a cerebrovascular accident (CVA), is aphasic. We are seeing him in a nursing home. He is now able to communicate quite adequately except in talking situations, where he becomes emotional. When this occurs, he cannot use the methods we have taught him to recall the names of things. This creates problems in the dining room of the nursing home because he is unable to order food from the menu. This S− situation must be dealt with, not only for the emotional state of the client but also to eliminate the problem in the dining room.

We would address this problem by getting a menu from the dining room and doing some role playing in the clinic room. Because we and the clinic room are both S+, the probability that the client can successfully order from the menu is quite high. We first sit with the client and decide on what he would like to order from the menu. The order is rehearsed with the client so he is familiar with what he is going to say. We then seat the client at a table in the clinic room and walk up to him as the waiter would do in the dining room. We hand him the menu and ask for his order. This arrangement is worked through until he is secure in ordering from us. We then bring in another person and repeat the situation until he can order from this person. His confidence in ordering from the menu is strengthened, and this reduces the amount of anxiety associated with ordering in the dining room.

Example 2. We are working with a 35-year-old man who stutters. His job calls for him to do a great deal of dictating, but he finds that when he picks up the microphone to dictate, his level of anxiety increases to the point where he cannot use the new speech behaviors we have taught him. The dictating equipment plays a strong S− role that we need to deal with in the clinical environment. We do not have a dictating machine available, so we ask the client to bring the microphone with him when he comes in for therapy.

We start our role shift of the dictating machine by having the client dictate a letter while looking at the microphone that is placed on the table directly in front of him. When he can do this while using the new speech behaviors we have taught him, we have him dictate a letter while holding the microphone in his hand at his side. The next step is dictating while holding the microphone in his hand, which is resting on the arm of the chair. The situation is then repeated with the microphone held to the side of the face. Finally, we have the client dictate with the microphone held directly in front of his mouth. We have not directly worked with the dictating machine, but we have reduced the S− role of the microphone, and this should increase the probability that the client will be able to use the new speech behaviors while dictating in the office. We might also suggest to the client that he not look at the dictating machine while dictating. If he looks only at the microphone, he will be better able to use his new speech behaviors, since the microphone is no longer an S−.

Planning and Problem Solving

The following clinical situations will present some problems for you to resolve. Think these through carefully, remembering in what stage of therapy we are. Make notes of your methods of dealing with the situations; then turn to Appendix D for my discussion of the clinical situations. Again, there are many ways of dealing with clinical problems, and your solution may actually be better than mine (heaven forbid).

Situation A

Your client is a 50-year-old man with aphasia. You have established a very basic vocabulary. However, you find that when you remove the gestural guidance prompt for the water, the client will not produce it. You now have a situation where the sequence of events is the prompt, the response, and the reward. You do not want to remove the reward at this time because you want to reward the spontaneous production of the word. How would you wean the client from the prompt?

Situation B

Your client is a 13-year-old boy with cerebral palsy. You have been working on the [g] sound using a token economy. As you begin to reward every other appropriate sound production, the sound begins to deteriorate. When you go back to a constant reward schedule, the sound is stable, but as soon as you move from the 1:1 ratio to a 2:1 ratio, the sound production falters. How can you remove the tokens while maintaining the correct production of the sound?

Situation C

Your client is a 15-year-old boy who came to you with a pitch problem. You have succeeded in lowering the pitch in the clinic room, but the client tells you that he is afraid to use the new pitch with his peers since it is so different. He also reports that he is so tense when he is with his peers that he cannot even produce the new pitch. It is your decision that this situation should be at least partially dealt with in the clinical environment. How would you do this?

CHAPTER

9

GENERALIZING THE NEW BEHAVIOR

◆ Synopsis

The new behavior is stable and habituated in the clinical environment but must now be transferred to other environments. The generalization process is a complex one and often the most difficult phase of therapy. It is in this phase that we will extend the clinical process and the Clinical Interaction Model (CIM) to our client's external environments. If we have significant others available who will work with us, we must train them to assist us and teach them how to use their interactions with the client in a home program. If no significant others are available, we must compensate for their absence. All these issues are discussed in this chapter.

Antecedent and Contingent Events in the CIM

We are now at that point in the clinical process where the new behavior is habituated in the clinical environment. Our clinical task shifts to the transfer, or generalization, of the new behavior to other environments. We most often refer to this part of treatment as *carryover*. In my experience, this is the most difficult and time consuming part of a treatment program. I may have spent as much as 4 weeks of therapy creating and habituating the new behavior in the clinical environment, and then I must spend another 12 weeks or more establishing and habituating the behavior in the client's external environments.

Because we cannot actually be with our clients in their external environments, we must depend on other factors to get the behavior to occur outside the clinic room. With many clinicians, the only factor they appear to depend on is the habit strength of the new behavior. They feel that if the new speech habit is strong enough, the new behavior will occur spontaneously in other environments. This process may succeed, but unfortunately it is a slow and unpredictable process, particularly with younger clients who do not have approach motivation to change their speech behaviors. If a client comes to us because he wants to change his communicative behaviors, we have built-in approach motivation. But what about those clients who are sent to us?

We were able to create artificial approach motivation and/or avoidance motivation for these clients within the clinical environment, but we are now faced with creating approach motivation and/or avoidance motivation to generalize the behavior in external environments. The level of difficulty of this task is dependent on our influence on the significant others in those environments, as well as their availability and/or interest in the client's treatment. In order to increase the efficiency of the program and to generalize the new behavior to environments other than the clinic room, we need a more specific program that, if possible, should include the client's significant others. We develop such a program in the remainder of this chapter.

As we shift the focus of our treatment to environments other than the clinic room, the contingent events continue to be important. However, we will concentrate on the antecedent events; that is, the stimuli that have assumed specific roles in the client's life (conditioned stimuli). These stimuli include the significant others in the client's life, talking situations the client experiences, and objects the client associates with communication. We must recognize that the client has already established talking habits in response to these stimuli. The stimuli cue specific speech behaviors. The client has talked "incorrectly" to the significant others in his life for a lengthy period of time. The significant others have either rewarded his incorrect speech by listening to him and responding to him or penalized his speech by criticizing him. In this way the significant others assumed either the $S+$ or $S-$ role for the incorrect speech.

The talking situations also may have assumed stimulus roles. If a client has talked incorrectly in the home for an extended period of time, the home can become either an $S+$ or an $S-$, depending on the response he receives for his speech in this environment. If he has talked incorrectly in the home for several years and has been rewarded for it, the home environment assumes the S+ role for the incorrect speech and cues it to occur. Talking situations often assume negative stimulus roles (S−), particularly for the client who stutters. If the client is penalized for his stuttering when talking in front of a class, this speaking situation becomes an S−, cuing the client such that if he talks in front of a group he will be penalized.

Objects in the client's life such as the telephone and other objects associated with communication may have also assumed a stimulus role. If they have assumed an S+ role for the incorrect behavior, this could create problems for us as we attempt to discourage the use of the incorrect behavior. In other instances, the objects might have an S role, causing negative emotions that prevent the new behavior from occurring. These stimulus roles are an important factor that must be considered as we attempt to generalize the new behavior.

Stimulus manipulation was an important part of the previous steps in the clinical process. In generalization, it is our main clinical tool. We have shifted the roles of the significant others in previous steps and even dealt with some talking situations and objects in the habituation step. We are now going to devote all our attention to stimulus manipulation. The new behavior is now occurring on a predictable basis, but it is not occurring with all of the appropriate stimuli. It is too restricted. We must generalize it so that it occurs when outside stimuli are present.

The clinician's clinical tasks change drastically in this step of therapy. The behavior is occurring naturally in the clinical environment, so clinical rewards and penalties are no longer necessary. Now the clinician's task is to orchestrate the client's external environments so that he receives rewards for the correct speech behavior and penalties for the incorrect behavior in these environments. This orchestration is accomplished through stimulus manipulation. The degree to which we can use the methods of manipulation will depend on the availability and cooperation we receive from the significant others in the external environments. Not only must the clinician carefully orchestrate the environments, she must also monitor them carefully so that, if necessary, environmental adjustments can be made.

Stimulus Manipulation

As we discuss the various methods of stimulus manipulation, we will change the order of presentation from previous chapters because we now have different clinical tasks, and the order of importance has changed.

Increase the Number of Stimuli

Our clinical goal in this step of treatment is to increase the number of S+ that cue the new speech behavior to occur. Thus far in therapy, the client has had only two S+: the clinician and the clinical environment. Where are we going to find the stimuli to add to the stimuli in the client's external environments? We are going to take S− and S0 and change them to S+. We started shifting the roles of other stimuli in the habituation step, but now this becomes our main clinical task.

Role Shift: Significant Others. We have been shifting the roles of the significant others as we progressed through our treatment. We are now at the stage where the significant others follow the pattern of the clinician in the habituation phase. In essence, the significant others are first habituating the new behavior in their environment and then generalizing it to still other environments. Early in the generalization of the new behavior, the significant others are very strong S+, rewarding every occurrence of the new behavior. These are the strongest and most stable S+ we are going to have in the external environment, so we must shift them carefully and make certain that the S+ roles are maintained in the early stages of generalizing the behavior. We will shift them again later after the behavior is stable in the external environment, but for now the stronger the better. This shift is seen in Figure 9.1.

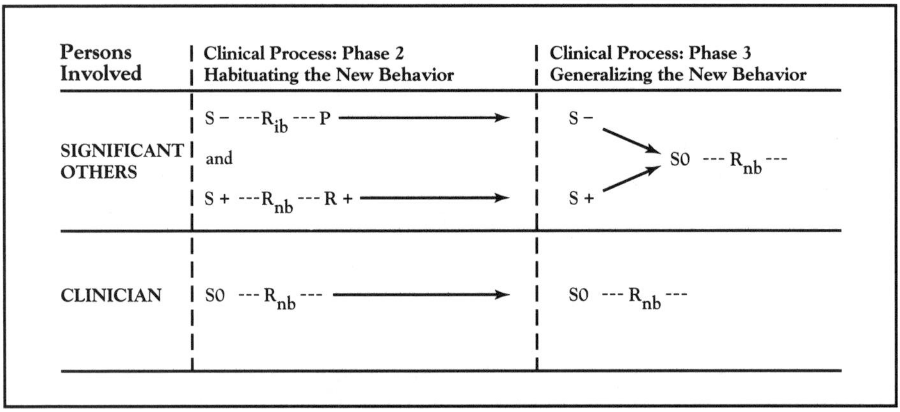

Figure 9.1. Stimulus role shift model—Clinical process: Phase 3. When the treatment program moves into Phase 3, the significant others gradually shift their stimulus roles from S+ and S− to that of S0, testing the habituation of the new behavior in the external environment by removing the reward. In that the new behavior remains stable in the clinical environment, the clinician maintains her S0 role.

Role Shift: Talking Situations and Objects. We need to assess the talking situations and objects in our client's external environment in order to determine if any of them have an S− role. This is particularly true for those clients who stutter, but it is also a consideration with any client whose negative emotions might interfere with the performance of the new behavior. When we discover talking situations or objects that have an S− role, we want to try to shift them to an S+ by associating them with rewards. If we cannot shift them to an S+, we want at least to neutralize their influence on the occurrence. We can shift them to an S0 by removing the penalty, but manipulating the contingent event associated with a talking situation or an object is much more difficult than working with significant others. We do not have the same degree of control over these stimuli that we have with the significant others. In order to make this shift, we have to use some other stimulus manipulation techniques.

As we discuss these techniques, let us not forget that the new behavior is occurring in the clinical environment. We are not discussing the performance of a new behavior for the client; rather, the performance of a newly *acquired* behavior in a variety of situations outside the clinical environment. If we are attempting to get the new behavior to occur in a talking situation that has an S− role, we may have to gradually introduce the stimuli. We are using the same procedures, except we do not have direct control over the situation because it is occurring in another environment. We must now depend on significant others to arrange the situation so that there is a gradual buildup of the stress in the situation, or we must depend on the client himself to approach the talking situation or the object in steps. We might tell the client who stutters to practice his new speech behavior on the telephone with friends, then with acquaintances, and then with business contacts. The client would then be gradually presenting the S− object to himself.

Another technique we can use is the gradual withdrawal of the stimulus. In this instance, we are talking about the significant others being the stimulus we are going to gradually withdraw. If a talking situation cannot be gradually presented, we may want the significant others to accompany the client into the situation. We now have an S+ (significant others) associated with the S− situation. If the significant others accompany the client, the probability of the new behavior occurring in the situation is greatly enhanced. The gradual withdrawal is then accomplished by having the significant others diminish their influence in the situation. For example, the significant others might actually accompany the client into a store while he interacts with the clerk. The next time the situation arises, the significant others wait at the next counter; they then wait at the door to the store. In this way they are gradually withdrawing their S+ influence as the client succeeds on his own.

Not all our clients have S− situations. However, for those who do, such as stutterers and aphasics, it is crucial that the clinician orchestrate the environment so that the client succeeds in using his new speech behavior in these threatening talking situations.

Decrease the Number of Stimuli. Here we are interested in decreasing the number of S− in the client's external environment. We accomplish this as we increase the number of S+ through role shifting. However, there is an important exception to this—we are actually increasing the number of S− as we shift the roles of the significant others to S− for the incorrect behavior. This is a highly controlled role shift. We are doing this so we can discourage the performance of the incorrect behavior in the most important external environment, usually the home.

We use all of the stimulus manipulation techniques as we attempt to generalize the client's new behavior. Now let us go directly to the clinical process and see how this is applied.

Extending the Clinical Process

At this stage of the game there has been a major change in the clinical process; we are no longer working within a single environment. We are now working in two general environments: the clinical environment and the external environment. The clinical activities in the two environments are very different.

The Clinical Environment

The clinician is no longer working directly with the client's speech behavior. She now has new clients—the significant others involved in the clinical program. She has to teach the significant others how to work with the client in their environment. They must get the new behavior to occur in their environment, habituate it there, and then generalize it to other environments. At this point in therapy their role in all of this is very similar to the role of the clinician. Therapy is now done through the significant others, and the clinician becomes more of a consultant than a clinician. She instructs the significant others, following the same guidelines (the CIM) she used when teaching the client his new speech behavior. She is going to provide modeling, information, and guidance for the significant others. At the same time, she is going to monitor their attention to the learning process and evaluate how much they have learned. She will reward and penalize them in order to create approach motivation and/or avoidance motivation in carrying on the home program. Essentially, she is providing the significant others with a crash course in therapy. She will set up the programs in the external environment, but the significant others are charged with implementing them.

The clinical sessions at this point in therapy are divided between the clinician's monitoring of the client's speech behaviors and her monitoring of the significant others' program through their verbal or written reports. She will have to be extremely careful about the types and amounts of rewards and penalties the significant others are administering. She also must monitor the gradual fading of the rewards by changing the reward schedule. It is a tough job, but there does not seem to be any easy way to get new speech behaviors to generalize.

Speaking of tough jobs, what does the clinician do if she has no significant others to assist with the generalization of the new behavior? In this situation, the clinician must either find other people in the client's external environment who will help with the generalization process, or she will have to figure out ways she can do it. It is very difficult to find other people to assist us. If we turn to teachers in the schools, we must realize that they have their own teaching to do, and they are extremely busy with their own jobs. The same holds true in other environments, such as nursing homes or hospitals. These other people will often provide what help they can, but it is quite limited since they have their own tasks to perform. All of this planning, bargaining, plotting, and manipulating goes on in the clinical environment. This is the clinician's job at this point in therapy.

Now let us consider this question: How are things planned for the external environment?

The External Environment

We need to be more specific about the external environment(s) in this discussion. For most of our clients, the external environment we are working with is the home environment. Initially, this is where we want the new behavior to occur. From there, we hope it will generalize to all the client's other environments. It is impossible for us to work directly with all of the client's environments; however, as the new speech behavior becomes more stable and more habituated, it will generalize to many environments without direct assistance. Early in the generalization of the new behavior, though, we must provide as much assistance and support as possible.

There are four unique circumstances that we must deal with as we generalize the new behavior. We have clients who are highly motivated to change their behavior, and we have clients who have no motivation to change their behavior. There are significant others who cooperate with us and assist in the generalization of the new behavior as well as absent or disinterested significant others who provide no assistance (see Chapter 4). We need to discuss the generalization procedure in all four situations. We start with the ideal situation and save the worst for last. By arranging the discussion this way, we may be able to pick up some helpful hints from the easier situations that will help us with the more difficult situations.

Motivated Client: Assistance From Significant Others. The therapy in the external environment consists of three phases. We must first get the new behavior to occur in the environment, then habituate it in that environment, and finally generalize it to other environments.

Getting the new behavior to occur. In the previous step of therapy, we shifted the roles of the significant others to S+ for the new behavior and S− for the old behavior. The behavior should occur in the external environment if the significant others are rewarding its occurrences and the client has approach motivation to change his behavior. If not, we may have to work with the client with the significant others present in the clinical setting. When the new behavior occurs for us, we have the significant others give the reward. This is a more direct way of creating their new S+ role. The S+ role is important with this type of client, serving as a supplement to the client's own motivation. The S− role is of lesser importance because the client already has approach motivation. If the approach motivation lags as generalization progresses, we can still turn to avoidance motivation, but it may not need to be used.

We must monitor the significant others carefully in such a home program. All they know about the clinical process is what we have taught them. If things are so simple that you can train significant others completely in a couple of hours, why does it take so many years to train a competent speech clinician? Keep in mind that the significant others have no deep insights into why they are doing what they are doing. They are following your instructions.

If the new behavior is not stable in the external environment, the significant others may have to do some modeling. This can easily be explained to the significant others in terms of having them show the client how the new behavior should be performed. At most, this should be a short-term arrangement. The behavior has not been forgotten; it is just that the transfer of the behavior to the external environment is too big a step for the client. Some modeling with constant rewards for performing the new behavior should rectify this situation quickly. And do not forget, we have the approach motivation of the client working for us.

The most difficult task, I have found, is getting the significant others to maintain their S+ and S− roles long enough for the new behavior to generalize. They tend to feel that when the new behavior has occurred and been rewarded several times this is sufficient. I mention this problem here because I have had difficulty with some significant others maintaining their roles—even during this first phase of the home program. Giving the significant others heavy doses of reward for maintaining their roles seems to do the trick.

Habituating the new behavior. Habituation is accomplished just as it was in the clinical environment. We adjust the ratio of rewards so that the significant others gradually shift their roles again. We slowly withdraw the S+ and S− roles as the behavior establishes itself in the new environment. Again, we are testing habituation. If the new behavior begins to falter, the significant others must increase the amount of reward associated with it. As mentioned earlier, it is not uncommon for the significant others to tend to rush the withdrawal of rewards. They need to recognize that even though a behavior might be quite stable in their environment, it might be just starting to be established in other environments. It is much better to extend the reward system beyond its useful time than to terminate it before the behavior is stabilized. The significant others must be carefully monitored in order to maintain the gradual withdrawal of the reward.

Generalizing the new behavior. In most instances, once the new behavior is habituated in the significant others' environment it will naturally generalize to the client's other environments. However, in some cases the client's new behavior occurs in the significant others' environment but does not occur in other environments. These clients need a cue or prompt to help them remember to produce the new behavior when there are no S+ or S− in the environment. We must remember that in the other environments there may be talking situations and objects that have assumed an S− role. Other people, such as authority figures, may also have assumed such a role. This is where gradual presentation and gradual withdrawal of the stimuli come in handy.

As the client starts to generalize his new behavior to other environments, the significant others can use reminders to help the client. A reminder is anything unusual that, when noticed, reminds a person to do something. An example will make the idea clear. One client would turn over a chair in the middle of the kitchen when he wanted to remember something important. He would then come down to the kitchen in the morning and wonder why a chair was upside down in the middle of the floor. But it would remind him to remember to do something important, like make a telephone call. This worked very well for him until he came down to the kitchen in the middle of the night for a snack and fell over the chair in the dark. He broke the chair and his leg. He decided to change his reminder to a slipper on the bathroom counter.

Here is a list of some reminders I have taught significant others to use when helping clients remember to produce the new behavior:

1. An adhesive bandage on a finger
2. A string around a finger
3. Wearing the watch on the "wrong" wrist
4. A small adhesive dot on the side of the lens of the glasses
5. Carrying an unusual object in trousers' pocket
6. Wearing a ring on the "wrong" finger
7. Wearing a bracelet on the "wrong" wrist
8. A ball and chain on the ankle

This should give you an idea of what I use as reminders. Each of these things will last for only a short time. As soon as the client becomes accustomed to the reminder, it no longer helps. We must change these often in order for them to provide the cue or prompt for the client.

We can also use verbal reports from the client both to us and the significant others as to how well he is able to use the new speech behavior in other environments. However, there is a better way to obtain this information than to rely on the client's memory. We can have the client keep a logbook of talking situations where he is practicing his new speech behavior in other environments. The client should share his logbook with us and the significant others. Because the logbook forms the core of our work with clients when there are no significant others to work with us, we discuss the use of the logbook in detail in the following section. However, remember that the logbook can also be used effectively with clients where the significant others are working with us.

Motivated Client: No Assistance from Significant Others. We are sometimes faced with a situation where the significant others are either not available or not interested in assisting with therapy. Our first step in such a situation is to try to arrange to have other people in the client's environment assist us in generalization. As we discussed earlier, this poses a problem in terms of coordinating their efforts and making sure they are consistent in their rewards and penalties. It is also a problem to find another person who has, or will, take the time to help us. We should try to find people who can assume S1 and S roles.

Our first clinical task in generalizing the behavior is to select some external environment where we can concentrate our efforts. This might well be that environment where we are able to find other people who will work with us. If we cannot get assistance, we must work with the client to determine an appropriate environment. With a motivated client this is not a difficult task. We might decide on a work environment with an adult client or a particular classroom environment with a younger client. In any event, we should focus our efforts on a specific environment rather than use a shotgun approach; that is, instead of trying to work with all of the client's environments at the same time.

Once we have decided on the environment where the client is going to start using the new behavior, we must figure out some way of getting the client to perform the new behavior and a method for him to report his success or failure to us. This is vital information, because if the client is failing in his attempts to use the new behavior, we must change our approach so he can succeed. If we have no significant others to work with us, we cannot set up a structured program as we did in the previous section. We will follow the same general procedures, but since we have so little control over the external environments, we will need to make adjustments as we go along.

My most successful approach to this clinical situation has been with the speech logbook. This is patterned after the Stress-Inoculation Training (SIT) program by Meichenbaum (1977) for training in coping skills to dealing with stressful situations. Meichenbaum and Cameron (1973), in their article on training in self dialogue with schizophrenics, acknowledge rehearsals as part of the practice for newly learned language skills. Radnitz (2000) reports on self-report measures that are used in a variety of ways including evaluating symptom severity, frequency, and/or duration. These references support the concept of the logbook that follows.

I carefully explain to the client that the logbook is for recording his speech practice and his speech game situations. Practice occurs when the client is concentrating on *how* he is talking rather than on *what* he is talking about. During these situations, the client is making a very special effort to have the new speech behavior occur. It might even be necessary for some clients to memorize what they are going to say so that when the situation does occur, they can concentrate on how they are talking. Let us think of this in terms of the client's attention being directed 75% toward how he is talking and 25% on what he is talking about. A game is talking, such as in a conversation, while attending 75% to what is being said and only 25% to how it is being said.

I explain the difference between practice and games to the client by drawing an analogy with learning to play tennis. The coach provides modeling, guidance, and information regarding how to hold the racket, how to serve the ball, and how to perform the backhand. The coach then has the player practice each procedure independently. For the serve, the player stands at the line and serves 40 balls to the other side of the court. There is no return of the ball, just practice of the serve. For the backhand, the coach hits balls to the player in such a way that the player can practice returning the ball with the backhand. After several weeks of practice of the various moves in tennis, the player enters a game with another person. He will not be practicing during the game, he will be testing to see how well he has learned through his practice. He will find out, in the game, how much more he needs to practice and on what moves.

The logbook is primarily for recording the practice of the new speech behavior in the external environment. There may be four or five practice sessions each day. However, each practice session is quite short, since the client will find it very difficult to concentrate on how he is talking for an extended period of time. As the behavior becomes more stable in the external environments, the practice sessions can last longer. At that time, the client can also include reports on games (i.e., conversations where he attempted to use the new behavior).

The size of the logbook is also an important issue. It should be small enough to carry in a pocket, because the client must carry it with him at all times. The only times that the client may be without the logbook are when sleeping and in the shower. The logbook will not remind him to practice his new speech behaviors or record the success of its practice if it is at home on a table. I have the client purchase a small spiral notebook, with the spiral along the edge rather than along the top. You may not consider this important, but I can never tell the front from the back if the spiral is on top. I never know which way to turn the pages.

I have the clients enter very specific information for each practice session. First, I have them write down enough information about the practice so they can remember it when we discuss it. This is usually just a couple of words to remind the client what the situation was. Depending on the client, I might then have him rate his stress as he went into the practice situation. Talking situations vary in terms of the amount of stress. Speaking to a peer may be easier for the client than speaking to a group of peers, which might be easier than speaking to a large group of authority figures. As the client is put under more stress, the probability that he will be able to use his new speaking behavior correctly is diminished. Thus, if we can have the client record the amount of stress he is experiencing when he enters a practice situation, we can adjust our expectations. My clients rate their stress on a 5-point scale, where a 1 situation is the easiest and a 5 situation is the most stressful. I expect a better performance in a 1 or 2 situation than I do in a 4 or 5 situation. The scale also helps the client understand why he may perform his new behavior better in one situation than in another.

The client enters the first two items in the logbook before he goes into the practice situation. He has identified the situation and rated the situation's degree of stress. He now practices his new speech behavior. Upon completion of the practice, I have the client rate his degree of stress again, using the same 5-point scale. I have found that this is very important. If the client has had a very successful practice and was able to use the new speech behavior, the degree of stress in the situation will reduce. The client might go into a practice situation he rated a 4, but after a very successful practice, the stress is reduced and the client now rates the situation a 3. He is gaining self-confidence in using the new behavior. This is a vital component in the treatment of the aphasic, the stutterer, and other clients for whom there is emotional involvement in the disorder. Barlow (1988) addresses the issue of emotional involvement in disorders. Under the heading of "Exposure," he states that there are two types of exposure: direct, where the feared situation is repeatedly confronted, and indirect, where the fear is confronted symbolically. In the logbook, the client uses both types of exposure when the stutterer practices his speech for the speaking situation (indirect) and when he actually speaks in the situation (direct).

The next bit of information I need from the client is some sort of indication of how well he was able to use the new behavior. The easiest thing I have found is a simple grading system: A for perfect use to E for inability to use it. Yes, it is subjective, but at least it is some sort of indication of what is going on when the client is working on his own. In using the grading system, I must train the client to grade his speech. I compare his grade with my own, and we adjust his level of expectancy to mine. Essentially, I am calibrating the client to be a good judge of his speech so I can keep track of his success in generalizing his speech behavior.

The analysis of the logbook in the therapy session is rather detailed. Figure 9.2 presents an example of three log entries a client might bring in and how they would be analyzed for him.

The client in Figure 9.2 is an adult with aphasia who is in a nursing home, and this is the environment on which we have decided to focus. We

LOGBOOK		
Situation 1	**Situation 2**	**Situation 3**
1. lunch	1. nurse	1. phone
2. 4	2. 3	2. 4
3. 2	3. 3	3. 3
4. B+	4. B	4. B−

Figure 9.2. Three logbook situations.

worked on some of these talking situations and objects while we were in the habituation phase of therapy. His logbook reports that he practiced his new speech behavior (recalling the names of objects) in three situations. He ordered his lunch, talked to the nurse, and made a telephone call to his family. He indicated that there was a lot of stress in the practice situations of ordering lunch and telephoning his family, rating them as 4 situations. These ratings indicate that the client expected to have a great deal of difficulty in the talking situations. But the ratings he made after the practice indicated that he was quite successful and lost some of the fear of the talking situations. We had rehearsed ordering lunch, and he did a good job. His stress was reduced from a 4 to a 2. We also worked with the telephone, and this situation also showed a reduction in stress from a 4 to a 3. The only situation that did not result in reduced stress was talking to the nurse, but we had not rehearsed this. Still, the practice was very successful. He reported that his speech was at a Grade B level. The lowest grade he gave himself was the B− on the telephone.

The degree of success is reviewed with the client on a highly cognitive level. His success is strongly rewarded through verbal praise and pointing out carefully how well he did in using his new speech. The client's logbook is carefully reviewed in each therapy session, with a heavy emphasis on rewarding him for his success As the client gains confidence, the first rating of stress (Item Number 2) is reduced. The stress rating for ordering lunch is reduced from a 4 to a 3 to a 2, and so on. Eventually, the expectation of stress lowers to the point where it matches the actual stress experienced. This is a strong indication that some significant cognitive changes are taking place.

At the same time, the grades for speech improve. I compare the grades with the second rating of stress (Item Number 3). If the client has collected 35 practice situations in a week, I list all the grades for each level of stress. As the client practices the new behavior in the environment and gains confidence, the grades improve. My analysis might look like this:

(5) D, D, D+
(4) D+, C−, C, C+, C+
(3) C−, C, C, C+, C+, B, B
(2) C, C, C+, C, C+, B, B−, B, B+
(1) B−, B, B−, B, B, B+, B+, A−, B+, A−, A

Your records may not look this good, but the point is that the grades will improve over time. As I analyze the two situations, for example, I might point out to the client that the week started with grades of C for the new speech behavior, but that after nine practices during the week, he had raised the grade up to a B+. I would give a lot of verbal praise for raising the grade that much in only 1 week.

We must remember that in this clinical situation, where we have a motivated client but no significant other involvement, the only active support the client receives is from us. We are his one and only support system. If we are trying to increase the number of S+ to encourage the new behavior to occur, let us look to the logbook. First of all, it serves as a reminder for the client to perform his behavior. It also results in rewards when we review and analyze it. Through this association with rewards, the logbook becomes a very strong S+. It is almost an extension of the clinician into the client's external environment, reminding the client to perform his practice and cuing the new behavior to occur.

When we had cooperation from the significant others, we had both an S+ and S−. The logbook assumes the role of S−. In fact, it assumes two S− roles. First, it serves as an S−, cuing the incorrect behavior not to occur, because there may be some penalty associated with this when the clinician reviews the report (although I do keep penalty to a minimum unless I find I must use the client's avoidance motivation). Our client in this example has high approach motivation, so there will be little need to turn to avoidance motivation. This does not mean that we abandon penalty, we only use less of it.

The second S− role the logbook assumes concerns filling a quota of practice sessions. If the client is required to report four practice sessions per day, there is a penalty if less than the quota is handed in. In this S− role, the logbook cues the client to do his practice sessions in order to avoid penalty. How much fudging do I get? Some definitely, but not as much as with a highly motivated client. Usually the client just says that he did not have the time to collect all the practice sessions requested. If I have requested four per day but the client is consistently coming up one or two short, I negotiate with the client. I adjust the number required to the number of sessions he has been able to do in the past. Now there are no excuses. He has set the quota.

The logbook is as helpful in therapy as the clinician wants it to be. The assistance the clinician receives from the logbook depends on the clarity of the data the client enters into the logbook; the frequency and depth of analysis of the data by the clinician and the client; and the appropriateness, frequency, and consistency of the rewards and penalties associated with the logbook reports. When used to its fullest extent, the logbook is the strongest tool the speech clinician has for generalizing new speech behaviors. It is even stronger than most programs where the significant others are giving assistance. But, you say, what do you do for children? I have used the logbook with children as young as 5 years of age. As long as they can count and write from 1 to 5 and from A to E, I can adjust the logbook to them. It just takes some imagination.

Now let us move into those clinical situations where we are working with clients who are not motivated to work on their speech.

Unmotivated Client: Assistance from Significant Others. This clinical program is going to be quite similar to the first situation, where we had a client with approach motivation and cooperation from the significant others. With the unmotivated client, we had to create artificial approach motivation in the clinical environment through the use of carefully selected rewards. We also had to use the client's avoidance motivation to avoid our penalties. This works quite effectively in the clinical environment because we have direct control over that environment. However, now we have to create the same artificial approach motivation and avoidance motivation in the external environment. Since the client is not motivated to work on his speech, we must give him approach motivation to achieve the reward and avoidance motivation to avoid penalty from the significant others.

We will follow the same home program that we used for the client who has approach motivation. However, we are now totally dependent on the rewards and penalties from the significant others for the client's approach motivation and avoidance motivation. We must be extremely careful in our instructions to the significant others. They will need more insight into what they are doing and why they are doing it than those working with motivated clients. The rewards and penalties must be carefully selected. The token economy is particularly well adapted to this type of situation, because it is mostly younger clients who fall into this unmotivated classification. They do not see the importance of changing their speech. The significant others must provide the approach motivation and avoidance motivation in the home environment through rewards and penalties.

Getting the new behavior to occur. There are some changes in program emphasis with the unmotivated client. We have to be very careful in establishing the significant others as S+ and S−. Because this is our only means of creating approach motivation and avoidance motivation with this client, we should not rush this step. Make certain that the new S+ and S− roles are firmly established before starting the generalization program in the significant others' environment.

We will also need to monitor the home program more carefully. We are not to the stage of maintaining the client's approach motivation and avoidance motivation because we must first create them. We have given special training to the significant others, so their reports to us will be a bit more detailed than those working with other types of clients. This detailed information allows us to make corrections in creating and maintaining the client's approach motivation and avoidance motivation.

There may, indeed, be more need for modeling of behaviors by the significant others with this type of client. They should understand what modeling is and why it is used. As the behavior becomes more stable in the significant others' environment, the amount of modeling can be reduced, but it should not be withdrawn too soon or too quickly. This is where our monitoring comes in. The reports from the significant others are very important.

In all probability, the therapy with the unmotivated client will proceed slower than with the motivated client. For this reason, the significant others will have to maintain their S+ and S− roles for an extended period of time. I mentioned that I had difficulty in getting the significant others to maintain their roles with motivated clients. It is even more difficult with unmotivated clients because progress in generalization is slower. Do not forget to reward the significant others for all of the assistance they are giving you. This is a good way to maintain their roles. And, if you are clever enough, you can also work in some penalty.

Habituating the new behavior. There is really no change in the habituating procedure from that of the motivated client. I would only caution that the process cannot be rushed. It is slower than with motivated clients, and we must accept this, directing the significant others accordingly. We are faced with an interesting problem here. How do we determine if our generalization is going too slowly or if we are moving too fast? As in love and war, there are no rules. This is a professional judgment on our part and comes with experience. That said, if a clinician takes 2 years to generalize a sound into a client's external environment, this is hard to justify. Perhaps you can use as a guideline the old saying, "Let your conscience be your guide."

Generalizing the new behavior. The most radical change in this phase of generalization is in the use of reminders. Because the client is unmotivated and because there is no specific reward associated with the reminder, the reminders have little if any effect. How can we correct the situation? We can start by shifting focus to the logbook with a strong reward program. Even though the client is not interested in working on his speech, we provide him with approach motivation to achieve the reward. We use the logbook to keep track of how many rewards he receives. If he has approach motivation to achieve the reward, we can use his avoidance motivation to avoid losing the reward. Let us not forget that the significant others are cooperating with us in our therapy. It is important that we have the client share the logbook with the significant others so they can provide support through rewards.

We are also going to have to provide some direct assistance to this client as we attempt to generalize the new behavior to other environments, including talking situations and objects that make the client uncomfortable. Since the significant others are cooperating with us and have assumed the S+ role, it is important that they assist the client in transferring the behavior outside the significant others' environment. They can use gradual presentation and gradual withdrawal of the stimuli as an aid.

This step in generalizing the behavior with this type of client is exceptionally difficult since neither the clinician nor the significant others have direct control over the other environments. Careful monitoring of the significant others' program is crucial, and significant others need all the guidance that the clinician can give them. After all, they are doing the clinician's work.

Unmotivated Client: No Assistance from Significant Others. Now we have reached the most difficult of all clinical tasks. We were able to deal with this client in the clinical environment, because we had direct control over the rewards and penalties. We created approach motivation and avoidance motivation in the clinic room, but now we must transfer the behavior to other environments. Who can we turn to for help? We might try to find people in the client's external environments who would be willing to help, but this approach is extremely limited because it is difficult to control consistency and coordination. Furthermore, keep in mind that we have a client who is not interested in changing his speech.

The only things that we can use are rewards and penalties. We have assumed the S+ and S− roles, but it is very difficult to get other people to assume these roles. They may not be in contact with the client often enough or long enough to assume the roles. Also, they may not be consistent enough for the role to "take." This does not mean, however, that we should not try to get other people to assume the S+ and S− roles. With this type of client, we need all the help we can get. We should also recognize that it is going to be difficult to establish and maintain the behavior.

The most important thing we must do is maintain the approach motivation and avoidance motivation that we have established with the client in the clinic room. The rewards and penalties used there had to be appropriate, or we could not have created the approach motivation and avoidance motivation in the client. We now apply these as the client takes the new behavior outside. What is the best way to do this? I have found that the best tool I have available is the logbook. I can manipulate the logbook so that it becomes an S+ and an S− in the external environments. As long as the rewards and penalties are appropriate, the logbook will assist in the generalization of the new speech behavior.

With younger clients, with whom the logbook cannot be used, the clinician must devise some other way for the client to report on outside practice so that there can be rewards and penalties. We have to maintain the approach motivation and avoidance motivation we created in the clinic room, and we cannot stop rewarding and penalizing when the client is generalizing the behavior to other environments. If a logbook is not practical, perhaps a reward book could be used. We must devise something so the client can keep track of how well he is doing.

Is it best to establish a single external environment where the client will be expected to perform the new speech behavior? Yes. This is important so the client can initially direct his efforts to a single environment and so the clinician can plan the generalization program in this restricted environment. As the new behavior stabilizes in this environment, other environments (including talking situations) can be added to the practice situations in the logbook. We must make the process simple enough so we can exert as much control as possible over the external environment, and yet not so simple that the client is not challenged.

Can we try to establish approach motivation and avoidance motivation in this client through a cognitive approach? It certainly will not hurt to try. As we said earlier, we can use all the assistance we can find. If the client is an adult, we can approach him either intellectually or emotionally. We can set forth facts and other data, or we can make an emotional appeal. There is no denying that attitudes, emotions, feelings, and other such factors influence therapy. They must be dealt with when they are interfering with clinical progress. This aspect of therapy is discussed in detail in Chapter 11.

You will note that this is the shortest discussion of the four clinical situations, even though it is the most difficult situation to deal with. The reason for this is the limited resources we have when faced with this situation. But, as I said earlier in the chapter, perhaps you have gained some insights into how to handle this situation when we discussed the easier ones. In most instances, because we cannot plan ahead for this clinical situation, we must improvise. I hope that the strategies discussed earlier in the chapter will help you when you find yourself with an unmotivated client and no significant others to help you generalize the new behavior.

Before we move on to our discussion of clinical examples, you might wish to reexamine Figure 3.6 in Chapter 3. We now have completed the clinical process, and the figure will be more meaningful to you. When it was first presented, it indicated where we were going in our discussion. It now represents where we have been and should serve as a quick reference and overview of the clinical process and the CIM.

Clinical Examples

Motivated Client: Assistance from Significant Others

This client is a 37-year-old man. He is a physician who has recently relocated from South America to the United States. In addition to his private medical practice, he is a lecturer at a university medical school. Unfortunately, his foreign accent is so pronounced that his students, as well as his patients, have difficulty understanding him. His wife does not have any accent, having been born and raised in the United States. Our client has avoidance motivation to change his accent because of the negative effect it is having on both his practice and his position at the university. We have focused our clinical efforts on modification of certain vowels that are either distorted or used incorrectly. He is able to use the vowels correctly in the clinical environment, where there are enough S+ to cue their occurrence. However, in other environments, the original vowel habit pattern persists.

We discuss the problem of generalization with the client and his wife, and the wife volunteers to work on the client's speech in the home environment. With our client's consent, we set up a home program in order to shift the wife's role from that of an S0 to an S+. Since we are working with a highly motivated, intelligent adult, we do not have to turn to a token economy. Our task is to maintain the client's motivation by providing him with a sufficient reward for successful modification of his accent. We instruct the client and his wife to set up a regular time each evening when the client can tell his wife about his activities during the day. We suggest that the talking period be held at a regular time and that it be limited to 10 minutes. The client is instructed to use the new speech behaviors he has perfected in the clinical environment during the evening discussion. Furthermore, we instruct the wife to reward his successful efforts. She is cautioned not to interrupt him in order to reward him, but to interject her rewards at the end of phrases or thought units. Her reward consists of verbal praise.

If the client uses a vowel incorrectly during the phrase or thought unit, the wife is to make a note of the particular word and have the client repeat it correctly at the end of the phrase. If there is any difficulty in saying the word correctly, we instruct the wife to say it to him, providing him with a model. By using this method, the wife penalizes the client for his mistakes by having him repeat the incorrect words. This has the effect of creating the S− role for the wife. We do not encounter any difficulty with this arrangement with this client because of his high degree of avoidance motivation.

The reward and penalty schedule in the home gradually changes as the client becomes more proficient at using the vowels correctly in this environment. We must remember that this is not a new behavior that the client is introducing into the home. He has the behavior in the clinical environment and we are simply extending it to the home. Eventually, the wife will not have to provide rewards or penalties, as the incorrect speech behaviors disappear and are replaced by the habituated correct behaviors.

Now we might have to extend our generalization program into our client's work environment. This would be very difficult in the medical practice, but our client's lectures at the medical school give us an opportunity. We ask the wife if she would be able to sit in on some of her husband's lectures. Because she is both an S+ and S−, her presence in the lecture hall should cue the new behaviors to occur and discourage the occurrence of the old behaviors. A highly motivated client such as this would not object to this type of arrangement (unless the school insisted that his wife pay tuition for attending the class).

Motivated Client: No Assistance from Significant Others

We are working with a 27-year-old woman who is a singer with a rock band. She eventually developed vocal nodes from vocal abuse and went to a physician for an examination. He referred her to us to see if we could eliminate enough of the vocal abuse so that the nodes would be absorbed. We determined that the main source of vocal abuse was the hard vocal attack, not only in her singing but in her everyday speech. When in the clinical environment, she can use an easy vocal attack consistently in conversations and singing. We now need to extend this new behavior to her everyday conversations and, we hope, to her professional singing. Our problem is that she has no significant others who will work with her in changing her vocal behavior.

Our best tool in this situation is the logbook. We instruct the client that we want her to practice the new vocal attack in specific talking situations in her everyday speech. However, we are going to have to make some changes in the types of information we want her to bring to us. We have her include the following information in her logbook: (1) information to identify the talking situation; (2) a rating on a 1-to-5 scale of the effort used in initiating voice; (3) a grade from A to E that reflects her success in using the easy vocal attack; and (4) if she failed to use her easy vocal attack, what factors were present in the situation that prevented her from using the new vocal attack. The logbook provides us with several important features in achieving generalization of the new behavior. Most important, the logbook assumes both an S+ and S− role, since it is closely associated with us. We carefully review the logbook during each clinical session, and this association is what makes the role shift possible for the logbook itself. The logbook cues the new behavior to occur and dis-courages the occurrence of the incorrect behavior.

Second, the logbook functions as a constant reminder because we have in-structed the client to carry the book with her at all times. She may see the book in her purse but decide not to use the next talking situation for practice. But she saw the book, and through its S+ role, it cues the new behavior in-creasing the probability that the easy vocal attack will occur.

Finally, when we review the logbook with the client, we emphasize her successful use of the new vocal behavior. We maintain a heavy reward sched-ule for her success in her everyday talking situations. This is very important because we are the only support system she has. She needs to have someone who is aware of and pleased with her progress outside the clinical environ-ment. The logbook is our only contact with our client's performance outside the clinical setting.

Depending on our clinical setting and the agency where we are working, we might even arrange to go out on some talking situations with the client. For example, we might take the regularly scheduled clinical meeting time, go to a store in the vicinity, and have the client talk to some of the clerks in the store. This would be very helpful for the client, since our presence as an S+ would influence the occurrence of the new behavior, and we would also be able to provide immediate feedback in terms of the success of the situation.

We still have not dealt with our client's professional singing. We could have her use the logbook during her rehearsals with the band, reporting her success in using the new vocal attack while performing. We might also con-sider going to one of her performances so our S+ role would have some influ-ence on the behavior. We could also have her carry her logbook with her as she is performing. The viability of various alternatives depends on too many variables to list here, but they are considerations we should make in working with this client.

Unmotivated Client: Assistance from Significant Others

Our client is a 17-year-old girl who stutters. She has been in therapy for several months and has made excellent progress on her speech. When she started therapy, she was not even able to say her name in a casual situation. At the beginning of therapy, she was highly motivated to change her speech behaviors. She did her outside speaking assignments and kept her logbook faithfully.

At this point in therapy, she is able to speak in all situations, but she is not using her speech controls to the maximum. Her interest in therapy has dwindled because she no longer has a severe stuttering problem. Whereas before therapy she was considered a severe stutterer, she would now be judged a mild stutterer. When she uses her speech controls, her speech is normal, and stuttering blocks do not occur. The clinical task is to create either approach motivation or avoidance motivation in order to generalize the excellent speech she can produce when she is controlling her speech. When asked if she wants to improve her speech in her external environments, she says that it is very important to her since she knows how well she can speak when she controls her stuttering. However, she does not have the approach motivation or avoidance motivation to work on her speech in the external environments. She does not work on her logbook or attempt to control her stuttering in her everyday speaking situations.

Her parents are very cooperative and would like to have their daughter use the controlled speech in all situations. They realize that she can speak normally when she makes the effort. We have a conference with the parents and the client and attempt to determine if a token economy can be set up. We look for something the client wants to achieve (a reward) or something the client does not want to lose (a penalty). During the conversation, the subject of the client's car is brought up. The client uses the car every day, and this is her major source of social interaction, because there is no public transportation near her home.

The client already has the approach motivation to drive the car. We can then use this source of approach motivation to get her to work on her speech. We select the home environment because, through the significant others, we can control it. We then set up the following token economy. During the time the client is in the home, the parents are to respond to her speech by either presenting tokens (rewards) for controlled speech or taking tokens away (penalty) for uncontrolled speech. We use both approach motivation and avoidance motivation in this economy. The client must purchase the use of the car each day; that is, she must have a certain number of tokens in order to use the car. To get the tokens, she must use her good speech when talking in the home. The parents give her a token for good speech, not after every word, but after a certain amount of time. This is the variable interval form of inter-mittent reward. We are rewarding her for controlling her speech.

We are also interested in getting the client to monitor her speech more carefully, so that she is aware when her speech is slipping and can make the ap-propriate corrections. In order to get this behavior to increase in frequency, we will have to reward her monitoring and corrections. We then tell the parents that if the client's speech slips into the stuttering pattern but the client makes a correction bringing the speech back under control, they are to give her two tokens. Her self-monitoring and correction is an extremely important behav-ior, so we are rewarding it even more than the controlled speech.

We now have the approach motivation to work on the speech because, if the client does not control the speech and make corrections, she does not earn the necessary number of tokens to get the car each day. But we also want to consider the consequences of the stuttering when it occurs. Because the client can produce both controlled speech and stuttering, we want to reward the controlled speech to increase its occurrence and, at the same time, penal-ize the stuttering to decrease the frequency of its occurrence. Our final in-structions to the parents are that they should remove three tokens whenever the client uses the uncontrolled speech and fails to monitor it and make cor-rections. We are then penalizing not only the uncontrolled speech but also the failure to monitor and make corrections. Our client now has a great deal of avoidance motivation to avoid losing three tokens for failing to work on her speech. In order to make up for this single failure, she must have three suc-cessful uses of her controlled speech.

As you can see, we are focusing both on avoidance motivation and ap-proach motivation, with the penalty being the strongest contingent event. We are penalizing the client for failure to use the controlled speech or to monitor her speech and make the proper corrections. Our rationale is that if we penal-ize the uncontrolled speech, it will occur less often. What does the client use in its place? She uses controlled speech.

Unmotivated Client: No Assistance from Significant Others

We are faced with a 4-year-old boy who has had his cleft palate repaired, but still has too much nasality in his speech. This effect is also present in the pro-duction of the plosive consonants, which are distorted. He was brought to us by his parents, who decided that their child's speech was creating problems for the child in nursery school. Although other children were mimicking him, the child was not aware of his speech difficulties and was not bothered by the teasing of the other children.

We were able to create artificial approach motivation in the clinical environment through our reward system, a token economy with numerous rewards. We also were able to utilize the client's avoidance motivation through a penalty system where he would lose a token if nasality was present. We were successful in modifying the speech and habituating it in the clinical environment. Conferences with the parents were difficult to arrange because both parents were professionals, one an attorney and the other a physician. During the few conferences we were able to arrange, the parents reported that there was no change in the client's speech in the home or at school.

When a conference was held to arrange a program to extend the new speech behaviors into the home environment, we were met with what appeared to be cooperation from the parents. However, after the program was instituted in the home, the parents found one excuse after another as to why they were unable to carry out the home program. There was no follow-through on the part of the parents and, as a result, there was no generalization of the new behavior. Our first effort to correct this situation was to have a lengthy conference with the parents, where we pointed out the need for their assistance in generalizing the behavior. Again, although they expressed an interest in following the program at home, the program was not instituted. We finally realized that there would be no cooperation from the child's parents, and that we would have to approach the problem from another angle.

If the client were older, we might be able to work with him on a logbook or work with him on a cognitive level to create approach motivation. However, because the child is only 4, our only good option is to approach the nursery school teacher and see if she is willing to assist us. If she is willing to cooperate, we can set up an extension of the token economy in the school where she would reward him for eliminating the nasality from his speech. We would use a strong reward program in this instance in order to create approach motivation in the school environment. Penalty would not be used in this instance due to the lack of control we have over the school environment and the teacher's lack of professional background in speech therapy. In order to institute such a program, we will have to meet with the teacher and identify for her both the speech productions that will be rewarded, and those with nasality and distortion of plosive consonants for which there is no reward. With careful monitoring of this program, we hope that the behavior will generalize to the school and, finally, to the home.

Our other alternative is to continue working with the child in the clinical environment and trust that the new speech behavior will eventually generalize to other environments because of the strength of the behavior in the clinical situation. As I said earlier, this type of clinical situation is our most difficult challenge, and it is not limited to children. Unmotivated clients with no support from significant others pose many clinical problems, and each must be dealt with in a unique fashion. There are just no simple answers to this problem.

Dealing with Behaviors That Will Not Habituate

We have now completed the clinical process, but we must recognize that it is impossible to deal with all communication disorders in this procedure. There are disorders we cannot dismiss as cured or as stabilized. These are the disorders that regress because the client forgets to perform the controlling behaviors, or situations in which the client just does not want to be bothered with having to constantly monitor and control his speech. There is also the factor of fear, which when strong enough, interferes with the client performing the behaviors necessary to control the speech. For example, clients with severe hearing impairment must carefully control their articulation in order to maintain intelligibility. If the client does not do this, the intelligibility of the speech gradually deteriorates until it is unintelligible. Another example is the stutterer who must use specific speech behaviors to reduce the severity of the stuttering.

This type of client poses special problems for us. We cannot cure them of their disorder; the most we can do is reduce its severity. So the person must go through life with the disorder, trying to maintain the reduced severity achieved during therapy. If we dismiss a 20-year-old stutterer from therapy with greatly improved fluency, he is going to have to maintain that new level of fluency for another 50 years or so. This is a long time to have to maintain control over a communication disorder, especially if he is not provided with a maintenance program. It is our responsibility to provide the client with strategies and techniques to help him maintain the gains he has made in therapy. For our discussion, let us use a client who stutters, since this is the most common disorder we will have to deal with in this vein.

If we acknowledge that there is no cure for stuttering, we must also acknowledge that one of the problems faced in treating the stutterer is the relapse or regression that is a common factor in all therapies. This means that when therapy is terminated and the client no longer sees the clinician, the speech fluency slips, and the stuttering returns to some degree. This situation usually occurs because the client is no longer performing the behaviors he was taught to control his stuttering.

This problem first appears in the habituation phase of therapy. Because new behaviors do not habituate for the stutterer, they must be performed on a voluntary basis most of the time. However, we must still generalize the behaviors even if they are still, for the most part, voluntary. The stutterer is taught to perform the behaviors in environments outside the therapy room, but the behaviors do not become automatic in all speaking situations.

It is this lack of habituation and generalization that poses problems for the stutterer. In order to maintain his speech at the new fluency levels, he must perform the behaviors that create the high level of fluency. Since the behaviors are not completely automatic—still functioning at the voluntary level in many situations—they must be consciously performed in many situations. When he fails to do this, his speech regresses to a much less fluent level.

The challenge of the speech clinician is to provide the client whose new speech behaviors do not become automatic with a maintenance program. The program must be practical and one that the client is willing and able to perform. There are maintenance programs that call for up to 1 hour a day of a variety of speech activities, which must be recorded and analyzed. This is not practical. No one could perform this maintenance program for more than 1 month, and most clients would drop it after 1 or 2 weeks. The program may indeed meet the requirements of the therapy program, but it does not meet the needs of the client. I will set forth some things I feel should be included in a maintenance program, but you will have to create your own program for the individual client.

Training the Client To Be His Own Clinician

The first thing we must recognize in working with these clients is that they will be in therapy for the rest of their lives, and if they are to be in therapy, they will need to work with a clinician. A lifetime of formal therapy is not feasible, but a lifetime of maintenance therapy is practical. The diabetic, for example, is on a lifetime maintenance program. He must receive medication each day to maintain his life and his lifestyle, so he is trained to administer his own medication. You need to train your clients to be their own clinicians.

After completing formal therapy, the client must know what to do to maintain his speech. He must also have some objective means of evaluating his speech proficiency as compared to his proficiency level when he was in therapy. When he recognizes that his speech is slipping, he must then initiate the maintenance program and bring his speech back up to an acceptable level. In this situation he is acting as his own clinician, helping himself maintain his speech proficiency.

The client cannot assume the role of clinician automatically just because he is receiving therapy. In order to train the client to be a clinician, we need to involve him in clinical decisions about his speech, discussions about his future clinical goals, evaluations of his speech performances, and the assessment of his clinical progress.

The CIM is the teaching mode during this interaction with the client. The client must understand the principles and the processes of his therapy so he can repeat segments if needed in the future. Most of all, though, he needs to be an objective observer of his own behaviors and to know how to deal with his denial system. He must be made aware of his defenses, especially his denial, so that he can recognize them when they appear. As a clinician, he must be able to objectively judge his speech proficiency and determine the course of action needed to rectify the problem.

Stimulus Control

Stimulus control is the most powerful clinical strategy you can include in your maintenance program (see Chapter 4). You need some S+ cues in the client's environment to cue the new behaviors to occur, and it is going to be important to use any significant others if they are present and willing. As long as they continue to reward the new behaviors, they will continue to have the S+ role. You will also have to create additional S+ for the client, and you should include some S− in your planning. When there is a penalty for performing the incorrect behavior, the behavior occurs less often. The carrot and stick approach must be built in here. And again, the client needs to understand the principles involved so he can manipulate his own environment.

Record Keeping

The client should keep some record of the performance level of his speech. For example, the stutterer might rate his speech performance each day, by grade or percentage, and enter this information on a calendar. This will keep the client aware of his speech performance on a daily basis. Another client might record how often he is not understood and asked to repeat himself each day. Record keeping forces the client to monitor his speech, and this in itself will help maintain the proficiency of the speech performance. (For record keeping information, see the logbook section earlier in this chapter.)

Evaluation of Stress

With most behavioral performances, including speech, stress decreases the proficiency of the performance. A person might be able to play the piano quite well for his own enjoyment, but when he plays in front of an audience his performance slips significantly. The client is also being confronted with stress— communication stress. He may have to speak in front of several people, or be under pressure to speak more rapidly, or respond quickly, or talk loudly in a noisy environment, or read something technical aloud. Communication stress varies according to the speaking situation. The client should understand this and not expect as high a level of proficiency in high-stress situations. I have my clients rate their communication stress on a 5-point scale, where a rating of 1 represents speaking in the most comfortable situation and 5 is speaking in front of an audience of 30 people. With the two ends of the scale established, it is relatively easy to determine the remaining points.

Tape Recording

A periodic recording of the client's speech in a social interaction is a very good way of objectifying the speech evaluation. There are very small tape recorders that the client can carry in a shirt pocket or purse. I suggest to my clients that they make periodic recordings of their speech while talking to a clerk, a waitress, or a fellow worker and then listen to and rate their speech performance. The client might resist this because it is quite frightening to face reality by listening to one's own speech. However, it is a very important part of maintaining speech proficiency and should be presented to the client in this light.

Special Considerations for Children

So far I have discussed the needs of the adult client, but children present some of the same problems to us. For example, let us consider the 10-year-old child who stutters and who has been dismissed from therapy with much-improved fluency. He may not have the cognitive skills or the objectivity to carry on a maintenance program. In this instance, you will have to train the parents to act as the child's clinician. It is their task to maintain the level of speech proficiency. If the level drops, they must be able to institute a maintenance program. In order to do this, the parents must be trained as clinicians, not to the depth of the adult client but well enough to understand and apply the maintenance program you set forth.

General Comments

There are no hard and fast rules concerning maintenance programs. There is little, if anything, written about this aspect of therapy, perhaps because we do not know what to do for maintenance. We tend to recognize its importance because of the relapses of our clients, but we seem inclined to blame the clients and to suggest that they simply return to formal therapy. However, if the client has a comprehensive maintenance program, they might be able to handle their own regressions and relapses. The aspect of the problem we do seem able to deal with is client motivation. How do you motivate the client whose speech proficiency is slipping to carry out a maintenance program? The only way I know is through data collection, so that the client is made aware that the speech is gradually slipping and might then do something about it. Maintenance is a very difficult problem and may explain regressions, relapses, and frustration on the parts of both the client and the clinician.

Planning and Problem Solving

Situation A

The client in this situation is a 67-year-old widowed man who has had a laryngectomy. He is retired and living alone in an apartment complex with many other retired people. Although he has done a good job producing esophageal speech in the clinic room, he is still very depressed and fearful about the effects his condition will have on his life. You are now ready to extend the new speech behavior to other environments. What are the problems you would face here, and how would you deal with them?

Situation B

Your client is a 14-year-old girl with an extremely husky and low-pitched voice. She is usually mistaken for a man when on the phone, and strangers react overtly when they first hear her voice. She was referred to you by her counselor in the high school. Your contact with the parents indicated that they were also concerned about the problems, and they came in for several conferences during your therapy. They discuss the voice problem with their daughter at home and send you reports on any changes in voice production at home.

You have achieved a new pitch level with the client that she can maintain in the clinical environment. At the higher pitch level, the huskiness of her voice is eliminated. However, the client does not use the new voice in any other environment. She reports that she likes the new voice, but it sounds so different from her original voice that her friends look startled when she uses it. She also reports that she is extremely tense when she is about to try it outside the clinic room. The tension makes it almost impossible to produce the new voice. What problems might you face with this client, and how might you deal with them in order to achieve generalization?

Situation C

This client is 65 years old and has had a stroke. He is retired and living at home with his wife. His main difficulty is in comprehending what is said to him. You have taught him strategies to assist him in comprehension, and he is functioning with no difficulty in the clinical environment and with his wife at home. However, when he is in situations where he is talking with someone other than his wife, he becomes so fearful that he will not be able to comprehend what is being said that he cannot tolerate the situation. Further, his high level of anxiety in these situations interferes with his ability to use his strategies to increase his comprehension, thus reinforcing his belief that he can never function outside the home. The new behaviors to increase comprehension are not generalizing to other environments. Determine what problems you see in this situation, and set forth a plan of action that will resolve the problems. Again, you will find a discussion of these situations in Appendix D.

S E C T I O N

III

SPECIAL ASPECTS OF THERAPY

GROUP THERAPY: THE SHAPING GROUP

◆ Synopsis

The Clinical Interaction Model (CIM) is not limited to individual therapy or individual interactions with a client; it also applies to group therapy. Group therapy takes many forms in our field, and some forms are more effective and efficient than others. The shaping group, a unique and new form of group therapy, has been developed specifically to emphasize the advantages of group therapy and minimize the disadvantages. This chapter demonstrates the differences between types of group therapy and demonstrates the strengths of the shaping group. Operational and procedural guidelines of the shaping group are presented so you will be able to create such a group.

Definitions of Terms

Over the years that I have supervised therapy, I have seen many forms of what is referred to as "group therapy." The term is applied whenever a speech clinician is working with a group of clients. I have classified these various forms of group therapy into three rather distinct categories: mob therapy, therapy in groups, and group therapy. Let us discuss each form of therapy so we can identify it when we see it.

When we discuss *mob therapy*, we will apply the OP Rule, since we know that this applies only to the other people we have observed. In this type of therapy, the clients form a mob, not a group. The mob runs the group, and the therapist is controlled by the mob. The theme of this type of therapy is "chaos." No one, not even the clinician, knows where the mob is going or the purpose of getting together. The mob interaction is impossible to follow, since there is no overriding purpose, and you can always tell when you are observing mob therapy because the clinician has a bewildered look on her face as she frantically attempts to control the mob. As the mob gets further out of control, the bewildered look of the clinician turns to panic and then to hysteria. Needless to say, this form of group therapy accomplishes nothing. Mob therapy is not all that rare among speech clinicians.

Therapy in groups is the most common form of group therapy practiced by the speech clinician, particularly in the public school environment. Partially due to the role models of teachers and students found in this environment, the clients are expected to play a passive role in the classroom as the clinician assumes the more assertive role. When the children come for therapy in a group, they behave as they would in the classroom. They sit and wait for the speech clinician to organize the group activities, decide who will receive therapy in what order, and make the decision as to the correctness or incorrectness of speech behavior. In other words, the speech clinician is performing individual therapy in the group. The clinical process applies directly to this situation because we are still in an individual therapy mode. The reason that the children are brought to therapy in a group is for the efficient use of the speech clinician's time. It would be extremely inefficient for her to have to go to the classrooms and get each child individually.

Group therapy implies an interaction between the members of the group. It also implies that the members of the group are directly involved in the therapeutic process, both in terms of receiving therapy and in terms of providing therapy. This form of therapy evolved from the field of psychology where treatment is provided by the group. The group interaction focuses on the sharing of problems and possible solutions. This therapy form is rarely used by the speech clinician.

A unique form of group therapy, the *shaping group*, was developed in the late 1970s. We will discuss this group therapy process rather briefly in this book, but there are two sources you can turn to for an in-depth review of the shaping group (Leith, 1979, 1982). First, let us contrast the shaping group with the more traditional form of therapy in a group (from now on referred to as a therapy group).

Contrasts in Group Treatment

Group Member's Activities

In a therapy group, the clinician is working with one client at a time. The other members of the group are, we hope, listening and watching the therapy. They are waiting for their turn to receive therapy. Supposedly, this listening and watching activity has some therapeutic value. However, Mower (1972) found that these listening and watching activities have no therapeutic value. The clinician provides the modeling, guidance, and information; makes all of the judgments as to the correctness of the individual's responses; and administers the reward or the penalty. There is little, if any, group interaction. If there is group interaction, it often means that the clinician has lost control, and we are back to mob therapy. The only learning that takes place is when the individual members of the group receive their individual therapy from the clinician. The model for the therapy group is seen in Figure 10.1.

In the shaping group, each member of the group is actively involved in the CIM. They are involved in providing the modeling, guidance, and information for each other. They also make judgments as to the correctness of the responses and apply either the reward or the penalty. There is constant interaction between the group members. In essence, members of the shaping group

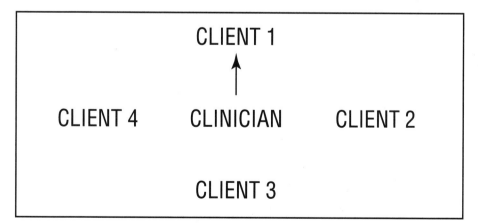

Figure 10.1. Therapy in a group model. In-group treatment with the clinician providing individual therapy for Client 1. Clients 2, 3, and 4 are watching and listening. This type of clinical activity is of questionable value (Mower, 1972). Reprinted with permission from Leith (1979).

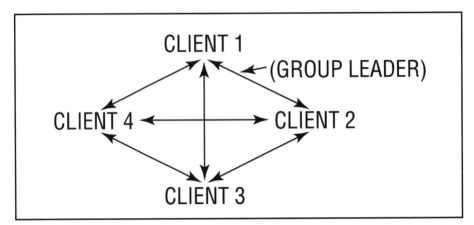

Figure 10.2. Group therapy model. The shaping group configuration with the Group Leader monitoring group activity, directing group focus, modeling appropriate responses to behaviors, and performing other tasks of the shaping group leader. Client activities consist of performing and monitoring new speech behaviors, rewarding or penalizing behaviors of other group members, participating in group discussions, and other forms of group interaction. Reprinted with permission from Leith (1979).

are playing two roles: the role of clinician when the group is focusing on another group member and the role of client when the group is focusing on them. Since the members are constantly involved in the shaping group, learning is an ongoing process for all group members during the entire meeting. Figure 10.2 illustrates the relationships in this form of group therapy.

Self-Monitoring Activities

In the therapy group, the clinician makes all the judgments concerning the correctness of the members' behavior. She teaches listening skills on an individual basis, and the only time the group member uses this new skill is when he is receiving therapy.

Group members in the shaping group are constantly involved in using their listening skills. Not only are they monitoring their own speech production, they are applying their listening skills to the speech of all other group members. One of the objectives of the shaping group is to teach all group members to listen carefully and judge the correctness of speech production. Self-monitoring is an extremely important part of generalizing the new speech behavior to other environments. The shaping group carefully teaches this skill.

The Clinician's Tasks

In the therapy group, the clinician's tasks resemble those we discussed earlier in individual therapy. The clinician does most of the talking, unfortunately, often to the point that the client cannot talk. The treatment mode has not changed; we just have some other people listening to and watching the therapy.

The tasks of the clinician change drastically in the shaping group. She is no longer performing direct therapy on group members. Rather, she is teaching them to function as clinicians through modeling, guidance, and information. The CIM applies here even though she is teaching behaviors other than speech behaviors. As the group members learn to function as "clinicians" within the group, the clinician assumes a more passive role, allowing the group to do therapy with a minimum of modeling, guidance, and information from her. She now spends most of her time monitoring group interaction and providing assistance only when the group needs it. The most difficult part of this new role for many clinicians is to be quiet and not monopolize the group interaction. Have you ever thought about how much the clinician talks in a clinical session in comparison to the client? Who is supposed to be practicing their speech in these sessions?

Individual and/or Group Therapy

With a therapy group, the clinician has no choice of therapy modes. She is doing individual therapy at all times. With the shaping group, the clinician has two distinct modes of therapy: individual therapy with a client or the shaping group process. The question that arises is when should she use each mode. Let us turn back to our five steps in treatment: evaluation, determining the behavior change goal, getting the behavior to occur, habituating the behavior, and generalizing it. The first two steps are not involved in the clinical process, so we now have to decide where to introduce the shaping group into the final three steps in treatment. It is probably more efficient to work individually with the client in getting the new behavior to occur and then begin the shaping group at the habituation stage. This does not mean that the new behavior cannot be taught in the group, but this tends to be a therapy group rather than a shaping group. As long as the clinician is aware of this so that she can shift back to the shaping group after the behavior has been taught, there is no problem. This is discussed in greater detail when we address the issue of adding new members to the group.

Types of Shaping Groups

Due to the wide range of client ages and other factors, there are four rather distinct types of shaping groups. Each type has some unique features based primarily on the ages of the group members. The most convenient way to differentiate the three types of groups is to relate them to the group members' school level. Thus, we will discuss the *elementary shaping group*, the *junior shaping group*, the *senior shaping group*, and the *adult shaping group*.

Elementary Shaping Group

The elementary shaping group is for children between the ages of 5 and 11. Because of the lack of social maturity of children at this age, this group should not exceed three members. The range of ages in this group is also critical. If possible, there should be no more than a 3-year age range among the members; however, the maturity of the children will influence this range. The clinician should consider this factor when starting an elementary shaping group. The male/female ratio does not seem to be too important with this group, although it is an important factor in other group types.

Junior Shaping Group

The junior shaping group is made up of children between the ages of 12 and 15. At this age, there is more social maturity, and the group size can be increased to four members. This group can tolerate a 4-year range in members' ages. However, a factor that must be considered is that this is the age of puberty, and puberty has strange effects on otherwise perfectly normal children. The male/female ratio becomes very important in this age group. Only the clinician can determine how to mix such a group, and she must take into consideration the clients' ages, their degree of social maturity, and how they relate to the opposite sex. The junior shaping group calls for some careful planning.

Senior Shaping Group

Clients between the ages of 16 and 19 are appropriate for the senior shaping group. We have to limit this group to four members, not because of puberty but because of peer pressure and its effect on group interaction. In some instances, where the clinician has a mature group of clients, she may increase the size of the group to five. The range in ages of the group members is now a very important factor. Peer groups seem to frown on interactions with younger persons.

So if a group consists of three 18-year-old clients and one 16-year-old client, there might well be a problem with group interaction. The age range depends on the makeup of the group and is controlled by the clinician. Gender also rears its head again; the male/female ratio is very important, and an equal distribution seems to be the best way to handle the situation. As with the junior shaping group, this type of group calls for some careful planning.

Adult Shaping Group

Clients from the age of 20 on fit into the adult shaping group. We have finally reached a level of social maturity where we can increase the size of the group to a maximum of six members. The only limitation we have here is the ability of the clinician to deal with increasingly complex group interactions. We are also no longer concerned about either the age range of the group members or the male/female ratio in the group. This is usually the most stable of all the types of shaping groups.

Mixing Types of Communication Disorders

If we happen to be able to create a shaping group where all the members have the same communication disorder, we find that there are some advantages. If all group members stutter, they have a common bond, and because they all understand how it feels to be a stutterer, there can be a close interaction, with clients sharing feelings and attitudes. On the other hand, if all group members have a problem with the [s] sound, it makes it simpler to provide modeling, guidance, and information because they apply to all group members. Grouping clients by type of disorder has some advantages, but also some disadvantages. For example, a group of children who stutter might be a very difficult group to get interacting. They would shy away from penalizing the incorrect speech behaviors in order to get the new speech behaviors to occur, and they would tend to be quite nonverbal.

Does this mean that mixing clients who have different problems lessens the efficiency and effectiveness of the shaping group? No. It simply means that if the members of a shaping group have different disorders, the clinician must train the group members to recognize different speech behaviors. This is all part of listening skill and is related to improving self-monitoring. A client with a voice disorder can certainly make a judgment about language structure and respond with a reward or a penalty. The process is a bit more complex but still operational.

Activities of Group Members

The clinical process cannot operate effectively in the group unless all group members participate in the group interaction. This means that the participants in the shaping group must monitor the speech behaviors of other group members in order to respond with either a reward or a penalty. This is a major change from the client's activity in a therapy group. The shaping group members not only must know what the behavior change goals are for all group members, they must also know which behaviors are to be rewarded and which are to be penalized. This information is provided for the group members by the clinician as she identifies each member and what behavior he or she is working on. This is accomplished during the initial organizational stages of the shaping group and is the basis for training the group members to listen to both *what* is said and *how* it is said, all of which forms the basis of self-monitoring. As the self-monitoring skills improve, the members' speech performance in the group will also improve because they will be better able to judge their speech performance.

Because the group members have not had experience in providing rewards and penalties for others' speech behaviors, they will have to be trained to do this. They will learn this both through the information given to them by the clinician and through observing the clinician as she initially models the presentation of the rewards and/or penalties. The most difficult thing to teach here is the presentation of the penalty. It is not too difficult to reward someone for a good job, but it is difficult to penalize someone. This concept is best presented to the group members by explaining that they can help other group members by reminding them not to perform the incorrect behavior. The reminder is in the form of a penalty and, since no one wants to be penalized, they will remember not to perform the incorrect behavior.

The strength of the rewards and penalties is crucial to the shaping group, and their strength is dependent upon the participation of all group members. Because the members form a peer group, the rewards and penalties are very meaningful, much more so than a reward or penalty from the clinician. Because the group members are peers, there is strong approach motivation to achieve peer rewards and equally strong avoidance motivation to avoid peer penalty.

Finally, all group members must participate in group discussions. These discussions provide each group member with an opportunity to practice his new speech behavior in a conversational mode. Since the topic of group discussion will also change, members can use their new speech in discussing a variety of topics, some of which might well take on emotional overtones. This will afford the members yet another dimension of speech—emotionally charged speech—on which to practice their new speech behaviors.

Activities of the Group Leader

Many of the group leader's activities have already been alluded to in previous discussions. This new clinical role makes different demands on the clinician. She is no longer the clinician in an individual therapy setting; she is now a guide, a moderator, a supervisor. In a previous article on the shaping group that relates to the treatment of stuttering (Leith, 1979), 16 unique tasks of the group leader were set forth. In this chapter, we discuss some of the more meaningful ones. It is already apparent that the clinician must carefully set forth the rules and guidelines for the operation of the shaping group. During this time she must also identify the speech behaviors and the behavior change goals for all group members. Once the group process begins, she must also maintain a balance between rewards and penalties in the group interaction. This last task is important so that the clinician can maintain the approach motivation and avoidance motivation of the group members. As the shaping group progresses, she must make sure that the criteria for rewards and penalties change so shaping can occur through successive approximation. This will necessitate guidance of the group interaction and the provision of additional information to the group members. Finally, the group leader must be able to allow the group to interact without her constant input. If the group is functioning well, they really will not need her input. The amount of group leader involvement in the group interaction will differ according to the age and maturity of the group members.

Operating the Shaping Group

Instructions

In order to avoid mob therapy, it is necessary to provide some rules and regulations. The group members must be instructed about how the group will operate, particularly what they must do to be a member of the group. The most important thing to establish is that all members must participate in the group interactions. This is also where the group leader introduces the concept of presenting rewards and penalties. A difficult concept to teach, but one that must be established, is that behavior change goals are achieved gradually. The group members must understand that the new speech behaviors introduced in the group will be learned in steps, not all at once. This is the concept of successive approximation.

Identification of Behavior Change Goals

The group leader must present each group member individually and discuss carefully what the incorrect speech behavior is, how far the group member has progressed, and what the behavior change goal is. This is an essential part of starting the shaping group because the clinical process is dependent on the application of rewards and penalties to the appropriate behaviors.

Rewards and Penalties

The group must decide on what they will use as rewards and penalties before the group procedure can begin. The members must make educated guesses at what they would find rewarding and what would be penalizing. The group leader will be able to confirm their guesses after the group process begins by observing the effects of the rewards and penalties on the behaviors. It is very important that the group members themselves decide (with some not-too-subtle guidance from the group leader) on the rewards and the penalties since they will be the recipients. The rewards and penalties must be easy to apply, not take too much time, and not interfere with the group interaction. The best thing might be some sort of auditory signal, such as a hand clap for a reward and a finger snap for a penalty. Visual signals are difficult to use because if the recipient is not looking at the person administering the reward or penalty, they will not perceive it. (It is impossible to maintain constant eye contact with three or four people at the same time.) Token economies work very well here, since the tokens meet the criteria mentioned above, and the backup rewards are better able to provide the variety a group might well feel is appropriate.

Getting the Group Started

After all the instructions are given, the group members' behaviors are identified, and the rewards and penalties are determined, we are ready to begin the shaping group. Since we are at the habituation stage of therapy, each group member is able to perform the new speech behavior but is still very dependent on the reward. The clinician must make certain that the group begins with a strong reward orientation. She should start the group by introducing a neutral but interesting topic for discussion. She might then ask each group member to comment on the topic. At this early stage of the group process, she might have to provide some guidance to make sure that the new behaviors occur. And when they do, she models the presentation of a reward for the group members. As the discussion continues, she not only continues to model the presentation of the reward for the new speech behavior, she also rewards group members who start to reward other group members. The presentation of a reward by a group member is a new behavior she wants to encourage. She does this by rewarding it when it occurs. When the group members begin to reward each other for their new speech behaviors, the group is off and running, and the clinician can fade her modeling. The group members are now providing their own modeling. The clinician can then assume the role of group leader by monitoring, guiding, and so on.

If a penalty is needed in the shaping group, it should not be introduced until the group is operating smoothly. As group members become involved in the discussion topic, they may forget to produce the new speech behavior. This is when the penalty should be introduced. Remember, we only penalize an incorrect behavior when we are certain that the client can produce the correct behavior.

Variations in Group Organization

As soon as the group is stable, the clinician should train various group members to act as group leader. This works even with the elementary shaping group—give them a little power and they fit right into the leadership role. Once the clinician has a couple of members who can lead the group, several variations in the group organization that add to the versatility of the shaping group become possible.

In order to train a group member, the clinician appoints a particular member to lead the group. She then provides guidance as the new group leader learns to lead the group and gradually fades her role as group leader as she transfers the role to the new leader. This group member then provides a model of a group leader for the other members of the group. The process is repeated until the clinician has as many new group leaders as she feels she needs. She can now vary the group organization. This variation in group organization is shown in Figure 10.3.

If a member of the group needs some individual attention, the clinician can turn the group over to the new group leader while she provides the needed individual therapy. The group can proceed with therapy without the clinician being present. Of course, this procedure should not go on for extended periods of time, but most clinicians who use the shaping group are amazed at how well the group can do without them. This form of the shaping group is shown in Figure 10.4.

It is often wise for the clinician to sit back and observe the group interaction and the performance of each client. She can do this by allowing a member

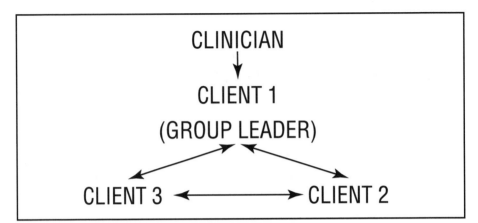

Figure 10.3. Shaping group: Leader training. The clinician is involved in training Client 1 to function as the group leader. The clinician assists the group leader in maintaining shaping group interaction. Reprinted with permission from Leith (1979).

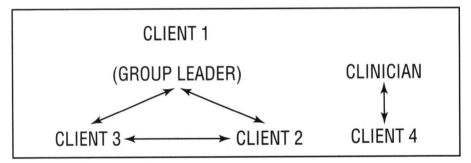

Figure 10.4. Shaping group: Individual/group therapy. The clinician is providing individual treatment for Client 4 while Client 1, acting as group leader, maintains the shaping group interaction. Reprinted with permission from Leith (1979).

of the group to lead the group while she observes. In this way, she can plot the progress of each group member, make changes in the group structure if necessary, and determine if the general direction of therapy is correct. This is illustrated in Figure 10.5.

Sometimes the clinician has too many clients to make up a shaping group. Let us imagine a group of six in an elementary shaping group. In this case, there are just too many children to make the shaping group work. So the clinician assigns three of the children to form a shaping group. She then assigns the remaining three children to serve as individual *monitors* of the three children in the

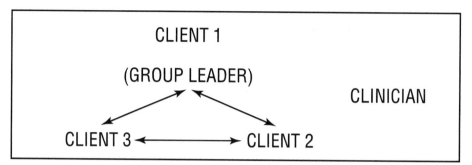

Figure 10.5. Shaping group: Clinician observation. Client 1, acting as group leader, maintains the shaping group interaction while the clinician observes and evaluates the group function. Reprinted with permission from Leith (1979).

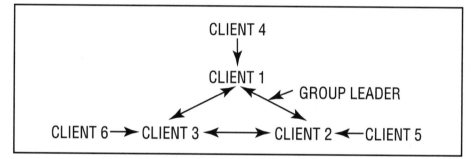

Figure 10.6. Shaping group: Group members and monitors. Clients 1, 2, and 3 are receiving a concentrated shaping group effort. They are receiving not only rewards and penalties from group interaction but also constant feedback from their individual monitors, Clients 4, 5, and 6. The group leader performs routine tasks as shaping group leader and also monitors the feedback among clients. Reprinted with permission from Leith (1979).

shaping group. The monitors' job is to sit behind their client and monitor his speech. They are to remind him to use the new speech when he enters the group discussion. They are also to provide rewards and penalties to their client. Although the monitors are not directly involved in the clinical process of the shaping group, they are learning listening skills and learning to monitor the speech of their client. This will directly influence their ability to monitor their own speech.

After a period of time, the clinician has the children reverse roles, with the monitors becoming the shaping group and the group members becoming the monitors. As shown in Figure 10.6, all six children are directly involved in therapy; they are not just spectators.

Adding New Members to a Group

Once a shaping group is in operation, it becomes an ongoing therapy procedure. Over a period of time, some group members will be dismissed from therapy. This does not mean that the group ceases to function. Rather, it means that we must add a client to an ongoing group. The new member has to be instructed as to how the group operates and who is working on what. This information is best presented by the other group members and can be accomplished in one clinical session. This is also a good way to have the group members remind themselves of the group's purpose and their individual responsibilities. The group then resumes therapy, and the new member learns to function in the group through modeling and guidance from the other group members. The process is repeated each time a new member is introduced into the group.

The Clinical Process and the CIM

If you go back to the CIM, you will find that it is operating within the shaping group, only in a more complex form. The stimulus, in the form of a question, may come from one group member. The member to whom the question is directed thinks about it and then responds. His response is then the stimulus for *all* the group members, and they evaluate it and respond. The strength of the rewards or penalties is increased because they are being administered by a number of peers. However, the strength may vary from time to time. If we have a group of four clients, they may not all agree that a behavior was correct. In this event, only those who felt the behavior was correct would respond. We now have the possibility of a range of one to three rewards being presented. Weaker rewards (those provided by one group member) indicate that the behavior is not as stable as it should be, while stronger rewards (those provided by three group members) indicate that the behavior is very stable.

As the speech behavior transactions continue between group members, the clinician also monitors the attending behaviors of the group members. She judges their approach motivation and avoidance motivation. If she finds a problem with either approach motivation or avoidance motivation, she can alter the rewards or penalties accordingly, or focus the group on the attending behaviors of an errant group member.

It is important to note that all members of the group assume special stimulus roles. Through the presentations of rewards they become S+ and through penalties they become S−. The group members retain these stimulus roles when they leave the clinical environment. If members encounter each other in another environment, they cue each other so that the new behaviors are encouraged to occur, and the occurrence of the incorrect behaviors is discouraged. In this way, the shaping group provides valuable assistance during the generalization phase of the clinical process. This is of particular value in the school environment, where the group members encounter each other during the school day. As you can see, the CIM extends beyond the clinical environment because all group members retain their stimulus roles outside therapy.

C H A P T E R

11

COUNSELING

◆ Synopsis

There are many instances in our clinical contacts where our clients, or even their significant others, have attitudes, emotions, feelings, or other cognitive sets that interfere with our therapy. As professionals, we should not only be able to recognize when these factors are influencing our therapy, we should be able to provide counseling for the clients rather than to ignore the problems or make a referral for professional counseling. Three specific approaches to counseling for the speech clinician are presented. It is just as important that when we do provide counseling, we recognize when we have reached our counseling limit and need to make a professional referral. We often find it difficult to make a professional referral because of lack of professional recognition by other professionals or their lack of interest. This topic and some techniques and procedures to use when faced with these problems are addressed in this chapter.

Counseling or Psychotherapy?

In most literature in the field of psychology, the terms *counseling* and *psychotherapy* are used interchangeably. I will use the term *counseling* in this chapter, but I do not do it to exclude the concept of psychotherapy. I view the differences between counseling and psychotherapy in terms of the depth of the interaction between clinician and client. Perhaps if we view this concept on a continuum, with counseling anchoring one end and psychotherapy the other, we can best understand the differences. In its most basic form, counseling includes such activities as giving advice to a friend, listening to a friend talk about his or her problems and then responding, or other similar activities we all participate in on a more-or-less regular basis. At the other end of the continuum, we have the most complex form of psychotherapy, used when dealing with severely disturbed individuals. I will not attempt to draw a line of demarcation between counseling and psychotherapy but rather allow you, the reader, to make this differentiation in your own professional life.

One of the issues that has confronted our profession over the years is whether we treat the disorder or the individual with the disorder. Our profession's origins lie in the field of clinical psychology, and our early professional training was closely allied with that of clinical psychology. During those years, the clinical emphasis was on treating the individual with a communication disorder. As the field of behavioral psychology became more prominent, we tended to identify ourselves more with the behavioral orientation, moving in the direction of treating the disorder rather than the individual. I suggest that choosing whether to treat the disorder or the individual with the disorder is dependent on the type of disorder with which we are dealing.

In this chapter, we will consider counseling a form of problem solving. We will consider those clients whose communication disorders have created problems in their lives and whose problems are reflected in problematic cognitions. With many of our clients, such as those with mild articulation disorders, their communication disorder does not interfere with their social interactions or their lives. However, with others, such as those who stutter or who have had a stroke or a laryngectomy, their communication disorder has created many problems in their lives. The latter group are the clients who need counseling to help resolve the problems confronting them.

I view counseling both as an integral part of our scheduled treatment program for some clients and as an augmentative program somewhat separated from ongoing therapy for other clients. For example, counseling might be an every-session ingredient in our treatment of a stutterer—building his self-confidence, altering his self-image, and reinterpreting his experiences of stuttering. Yet counseling might be only an occasional ingredient in treating an individual with a slightly deviant voice quality. This counseling might occur only when the voice quality has created a social problem for the client. Later in this chapter, we will also consider counseling as a completely separate treatment program.

The goal of counseling and psychotherapy is to modify a client's cognitive set, that is, the way they view themselves in relation to their environment and society, their self-concept, their self-image. Their view, for the most part, pertains to how they perceive their behavior in society and their own emotional reactions to their behavior. Their behaviors and their reactions to their behaviors are manifestations of their cognitive set, their beliefs about themselves, and how they relate to their social environment. Problems arise when the individual's perception of his behavior or his reaction to his behavior is distorted. In other words, the person sees normal behavior or reactions as abnormal, or sees abnormal behavior or reactions as normal.

Another way to view the cognitive set is to consider it as a belief system. A belief system consists of all of a person's beliefs about physical and social reality. A person's attitudes about his communication disorder reflect his belief system. If a person believes he is a victim of his disorder, his attitude toward it will reflect helplessness and passivity. His belief system will also include a number of beliefs about his social status, personality, and relationships to others. The belief system is the source of attitudes and feelings about behaviors that influence social interactions. The purpose of counseling and psychotherapy is to change the individual's belief system, to modify the attitudes and beliefs about his behaviors so he can see them in a different light.

Counseling by the Speech Clinician

Whether or not counseling should be included in our therapy is not the issue we face in our profession; rather, the issues involve who should receive it, who should administer it, and the intensity and the counseling approach that are to be used.

Stone and Olswang (1989) put it quite succinctly when they wrote, "There has been a lack of clarity about the range, depth, or style of counseling appropriate for a specialist in communication disorders." This is a classic example of understatement. One of the reasons for this confusion is the absence of any standards for training the speech clinician in counseling strategies. There are many questions that need to be addressed here, not the least of which concerns the role of clinical psychology courses in our training programs. If ours is indeed a people-oriented, helping profession, perhaps we need to reassess our professional commitment to the understanding of human cognitions, behaviors, emotions, motivations, and so forth.

We will approach the topic of counseling by the speech clinician from the three points brought up by Stone and Olswang: the range, depth, and style of counseling. Stone and Olswang deal with issues of the range, depth, and style of counseling from the standpoint of the boundaries of counseling to be provided by the speech clinician. They establish the boundaries by examining both the focus (i.e., the content) of the counseling and the interactional style to be employed. Let us discuss these points.

Stone and Olswang identify counseling that is within boundaries of the speech clinician's job, counseling that is outside the boundaries of the speech clinician's job, and counseling that is on the borderline of the speech clinician's job. Staying within the boundaries, the clinician can deal with the client's feelings and attitudes, problems directly related to the particular disorder, and problems the client might have with the treatment process. Counseling considered out of boundaries would include such topics as unrelated medical problems, chronic depression, and marital and domestic problems. These topics obviously call for expertise beyond that of the average speech clinician.

Topics the authors see as having questionable boundaries include those such as problematic, interpersonal relations between the person with the communication disorder and his or her significant others, a client's deep grieving about the communication disorder, difficulties the client might have in adjusting to the communication disorder, and behavior management of a disruptive child with a communication disorder. I do not feel that these particular topics are borderline for the speech clinician; the clinician must deal with these topics. Their importance is evident when we consider the problems faced by the stutterer, the client who has had a stroke or a laryngectomy, or the parents of a hyperactive child. And if the speech clinician does not do the counseling, who will? Who understands the problems faced by individuals who are communicatively disabled as well as the speech clinician? Who can appreciate the frustration and anger of a client with a stroke better than a speech clinician? Indeed, in my opinion, the only person with the professional insight necessary to counsel these clients is the speech clinician.

When working with the severely communicatively disabled, the speech clinician will be faced with counseling associated with the grieving process—grieving over loss. What have our clients lost? They have lost the ability to speak like other people. The five stages of grief associated with loss are denial, anger, bargaining, depression, and acceptance (Kubler-Ross, 1969).

The stage of denial occurs when the client actually denies that he has a problem or denies that his problem is as severe as it is. This refusal to deal with reality is a means of surviving, but it also stands in the way of therapy since the client sees no point in working on a problem that really does not exist. When a student receives a failing grade in a course, denial is often a means of dealing with the loss of a good grade. The denial takes the form of "There was a mistake in entering grades" or "It was a computer glitch." Everyone uses denial as a survival technique at some time in life.

The second stage is anger. Our clients are angry because they have lost the ability to speak normally. They ask, "Why me?" They are looking for someone to blame for their affliction. They are frustrated in their attempts to communicate. They are angry because they cannot say what they want to say or because when they say something people do not understand them. There is also a lot of anger directed to listeners who, in the client's mind, respond negatively to them when they have difficulty talking. The student who received the failing grade, also looking for someone to blame, is angry with the instructor.

In the third stage, bargaining, the client bargains in several ways. Some pray that the problem will be taken away in exchange for a commitment on their part to do something. One of my clients, a minister, prayed that if his stuttering was cured he would go into the ministry. He described the results of the bargain best when he said that both he and God lost; he still stuttered, and God had a stuttering minister. The client also bargains with the clinician. He bargains that if he faithfully attends all the therapy sessions, the clinician will assume the responsibility for curing his disorder. The student with the failing grade tries to bargain, offering to do extra work, to get his grade raised.

The fourth stage of reacting to grief is depression. The client, after failing repeatedly to overcome the disorder, becomes depressed. This is a common emotion with clients who have severe communication disorders such as aphasia, laryngectomy, and so forth. It also applies to students who repeatedly receive failing grades in a class.

The final stage is acceptance. The client finally accepts that the disorder cannot be cured. He also discovers that therapy can help him by reducing the severity of the disorder, perhaps to the point where it is no longer a major negative influence in his life. He then applies all the energy he wasted worrying about it to actively working on his speech in therapy.

Unfortunately, the client does not progress through these stages in an orderly fashion and then settle into acceptance. He constantly goes back and forth through the stages but, as therapy progresses, he spends less and less time in the stages of denial, anger, bargaining, and depression. Counseling will help the client move through the various stages as he progresses toward acceptance of the communication disorder.

I believe the most important factor involved in maintaining the professional boundaries surrounding appropriate therapy provision is the speech clinician's common sense. Perhaps there are clinicians who will overstep their bounds in counseling; all we can do about this is hope they will eventually recognize their limitations. This problem is not unique to our profession. All people-oriented professions face the same problem—professionals going beyond their level of expertise and counseling clients or patients in areas where they have no qualifications.

There is an old Arabian proverb that fits here. Read it carefully and see how and where it applies to you.

He who knows not, and knows not that he knows not, is a fool. Shun him.

He who knows not, and knows he knows not, is simple. Teach him.

He who knows, and knows not that he knows, is asleep. Waken him.

He who knows, and knows that he knows, is wise. Follow him.

I would add the following to the proverb:

She who knows, and knows she knows that this proverb applies to more than just counseling, has been reading the book. Pass her.

So how far should the speech clinician go in counseling? To the point where she feels comfortable with her knowledge about and insights into the client's problem (see the proverb). The clinician must not completely abandon her counseling obligations: She gives advice and counsel to her friends, so why not to her clients? If she truly cares about the welfare of her clients, her caring will prevent her from stepping beyond her professional bounds. She has more potential to hurt her client from the standpoint of omission than commission. Counseling is the manifestation of humanism in therapy. Without this, the clinical interaction is only mechanical, and the clinician could probably be replaced easily by a small computer.

With regard to interactional style, Stone and Olswang (1989) concern themselves with interpersonal relationships, power sharing, mutual respect, and other factors involved in the relationship between counselor and client. They do not address the specifics of the therapeutic process (i.e., the therapeutic approach). However, interactional style cannot be determined until the counseling approach has been chosen. The clinician must first select an approach to counseling with which she is comfortable, and this requires two decisions: what approach to counseling she wants to use and the type of interaction she wants with her client.

Counseling Approaches

The client's cognitive set may be changed through a number of different approaches to counseling. The clinician, depending on her point of view, has many choices of clinical approaches and strategies. The main problem here is that the large majority of counseling approaches are quite complicated and depend on the counselor having a rather extensive background in clinical psychology or formal training in the application of a specific technique. For a comprehensive overview of counseling for the speech clinician, I refer you to the article "Counseling Strategies for Communication Disorders" (Klevans, 1988).

The clinician must also decide whether she wants to use an indirect or a direct interaction. With the indirect approach, you allow the client to solve his own problems. You sit, listen, and nod. You may need to encourage him to expand on points and to reflect on his thoughts from time to time, but essentially you are a good listener. You can get field training in this type of counseling by going to a bar and observing the bartender counseling the people at the bar. You have probably used this form of counseling with friends who talk to you about their problems. This is an important way to start counseling, listening to, and understanding another person's problems. Establishing this kind of rapport will help you get to deeper issues that are troubling the person. This is a kind and humanistic way to start counseling.

With the direct approach, you are more active in the interpersonal relationship. You focus the conversation and direct it into areas that you feel are important. You ask direct questions and give direct responses. You advise the client with specific instructions. This is a much more efficient form of counseling because you keep the conversation focused on problem areas. This form of interaction is also more demanding of you, because with this technique, you are more active in the client's decision making. Your background in psychodynamics is more important here, but do not entirely abandon this approach feeling that you lack deep insights into human cognitions and behavior. A certain amount of insight is inherent in all humans. This is what you use when you do direct counseling with your friends, giving them direct advice on how to deal with specific problems.

We will restrict our discussion to three major forms of counseling: cognitive (dynamic), cognitive behavioral, and behavioral. The goal in each form of counseling is the modification of the client's cognitive set. In *cognitive counseling*, the cognitive set is modified as the client gains insight into his problems. The insight is provided either by the clinician in the direct therapy approach or by the client himself in the indirect approach, and this insight results in a change in the cognitive set. The cognitive set is changed in *cognitive–behavioral* therapy as a result of modifying the behavior that is creating the cognitive problem. New insights resulting from the modified behavior provide the means of changing the cognitive set. In *behavioral counseling*, the cognitive set is changed more directly through rewards applied to positive cognitions and penalties applied to negative cognitions. Each of these counseling forms is discussed below.

Cognitive Counseling

The steps in cognitive counseling are (1) focusing on the problem, (2) identification of the cognitive distortion, (3) confronting the problem area with new cognitions, and (4) changing the cognitive set through evaluations based on the new cognitions. We shall discuss each of these steps.

Focusing on the Problem Area. Let us use a clinical example to discuss this approach. Although the example and the discussion will be somewhat superficial, it will illustrate the points of this form of counseling. The example concerns a stutterer who feels that when he stutters, everyone stops what they are doing and looks at him. He will not order food in a restaurant because everyone will hear him, look at him, watch him as he completes his order, and then discuss him with the others at their table. He feels that he becomes the center of attention when he stutters. If the waitress stands across the table from him to take his order, he is even more intimidated since, if he speaks up, all the people in the restaurant will turn and look at him. This is the problem area.

Identification of Cognitive Distortion. The cognitive distortion is that the stutterer believes everyone in the restaurant will stop whatever they are doing and listen to him stutter. He also feels that they will discuss him when he is through stuttering. This belief is the source of a great deal of anxiety and fear for the stutterer.

Confronting the Problem Area with a New Cognitive Orientation. The new cognitive orientation is created by presentation of data and facts concerning people's activities in restaurants. It is pointed out that when people are in a restaurant, they are almost always interacting with the other person or people at their table. Their attention is focused on their immediate environment and not on watching the behavior of others in the restaurant. The tools the counselor uses to supply the new cognitive orientation are logic and reality, removing fantasy and emotional overlay from the discussion.

Changing the Cognitive Set Through Cognitive Evaluation. The changing of the cognitive set (belief system) occurs through objective evaluations based on the new cognitive orientation. The client is instructed to go to a restaurant and note carefully how the other diners ignore him. He is then instructed to order, noting that, even though he may have a stuttering block, the other diners continue to ignore him. Over a period of time, the cognitive set will change because fact and reality fail to support the paranoid belief that people are watching him.

Cognitive–Behavioral Counseling

In Chapter 3, you were introduced to the concept of cognitive–behavioral therapy. We now take these principles and apply them to counseling. However, the focus is now on behavioral performance and its influence in social interactions. We will use the stuttering client again in this example. The four steps in cognitive–behavioral counseling are essentially the same as for cognitive counseling, but now the focus is on behavioral performance as it relates to the cognitive process.

Focusing on the Problem Area. The problem area concerns the new speech rate the clinician is establishing to produce highly fluent speech. The client is pleased with the resultant fluent speech, but is disturbed by the slower rate of speech that he feels is abnormal. Because he feels the slow rate is abnormal, he is having problems establishing the new behavior.

Identification of Behavioral Distortion. The behavioral distortion is the client's misinterpretation of the speech rate. Measurements indicate that the new speech rate is well within normal limits. When the client uses the new rate, he feels the speech is abnormal, but when he listens to a recording of his speech when using the new rate, he recognizes it as normal. Also, when the clinician mimics the new speech rate, the client accepts it as a normal rate of speech.

Confronting the Problem Area with a New Behavioral Orientation. Having established the normalcy of the new speech rate, the new rate is introduced to the client's speech in the clinical environment. It is now easier for the client to use the new rate because his cognitive evaluation of the behavior has been changed and he now perceives the behavior as normal.

Changing the Cognitive Set through Behavioral Evaluation. The cognitive set (belief system) is now changed through the behavioral evaluation of the new behavior. Viewing the new rate of speech as normal allows the behavior to be performed more consistently, which leads to greater fluency. As the client hears himself speaking more normally, his cognitive set toward himself and his speech is changed to a more positive set.

Behavioral Counseling

In order to proceed with our discussion, it is first necessary to build a theoretical base to support our behavioral counseling. Earlier I used the "dead man" rule to define *behavior* (i.e., if a dead man cannot do it, it is a behavior). In this context, thoughts and feelings are behaviors. In the behavioral literature, these thoughts and feelings are referred to as *coverants*, a contraction of the words "covert" and "operants." We will use the term coverant to mean behaviors performed by the client that we cannot observe. We are talking specifically about the client's thoughts, his cognitions. The particular cognitions we are concerned with here are those that form the client's cognitive set: his emotions, attitudes, feelings, fears, self-concept, and self-confidence. For the cognitive set that is essentially negative in nature, we will use the term *negative coverants* (negative thoughts) in our discussion.

With some clients, the negative coverants will be an integral part of therapy. Our therapy must deal not only with the speech behavior, but with the negative attitudes and beliefs of the client. What type of client might have negative coverants severe enough that they need to be dealt with in therapy? Essentially the same type of client who would require deeper counseling, the client who has had a laryngectomy, the client who has had a CVA, the client who stutters, or the client with cerebral palsy. The list could be expanded to include any client who has negative coverants related to his disorder that interfere with therapy.

How do negative coverants interfere with therapy? There is an endless list but some of the more obvious ways are by distracting the client from therapy tasks, negating the client's motivation, creating deep states of depression or anxiety, and undermining self-confidence. If we are concerned about the efficiency and effectiveness of our therapy, we cannot ignore these negative coverants. We must include, as part of our treatment program, the modification of negative coverants to the point where they no longer interfere with our treatment of the communicative disorder.

Since coverant behaviors are learned, as are operant behaviors, they can be modified the same way. That is, the contingent event (reward or penalty) will influence the frequency of the coverant's occurrence. The problem is that coverant behaviors cannot be directly observed; their presence is only obvious as they influence associated overt behaviors. For the sake of clarity, let us illustrate this concept. A speech clinician has just parked her car in her agency's parking lot. She is getting out of the car when a man parking behind her bumps her car so hard that the taillight is broken and the fender dented. Does she become angry? Yes. An important factor I forgot to mention is that it is not her car; it is her boyfriend's brand-new car and he is a fanatic about keeping it neat and clean.

Now the question is, how does the other driver know she is angry? Anger is an emotion and a coverant. The emotion is manifested in operants that are observable and the operants reflect the coverant. Our speech clinician gets red in the face, she increases the loudness of her voice (that is, she is yelling), she restricts her vocabulary to shorter words (mostly of the four-letter variety), she stamps her foot, she pounds her hands on the car, and she exhibits other operant behaviors that reflect her anger. So operant behaviors can reflect coverant behaviors. This principle can be used to modify the negative coverants of our clients.

As our clients talk to us about their attitudes, feelings, and emotions, they will be overtly expressing their cognitive set, their inner thoughts. If we then reward or penalize certain thoughts, they will increase or decrease in frequency. Of course, we must be very careful with the type of penalty we use in this situation. The client might interpret the penalty as being related to talking about a negative thought, and the result would be that the client would just not talk about it.

The following is an example of a conversation with an adult who stutters where the principles of reward and penalty are used to modify the client's negative coverants. You can follow the interaction if you consider it as a series of transactions. We will follow the Clinical Interaction Model (CIM); the only difference is that the client's response will be the expression of an attitude, feeling, or emotion, rather than the production of a specific speech behavior. Let us consider a counseling session with a stutterer. As you read this exchange, keep in mind that this would not occur early in therapy, but only after the clinician had established good rapport with the client. You will have to imagine the client stuttering because when I wrote the counseling session and typed out the stuttering blocks, the text became too long for the chapter.

STUTTERER: I stutter so badly that no one wants to associate with me.

CLINICIAN: How can you say that? Didn't you tell me about your friend, Helen?

STUTTERER: Well yes, but she just pities me, feels sorry for me.

CLINICIAN: That's not a nice thing to say about Helen. You told me she was a very good friend and would do anything for you. Maybe it's you who feels sorry for you and pities you.

STUTTERER: I do feel sorry for myself. I have the problem with stuttering that I can't do anything about.

CLINICIAN: You sure are negative today. What do you mean you can't do anything about your stuttering. Are you saying you haven't gained any control over your stuttering during your therapy? What have you learned in therapy?

STUTTERER: I've learned to talk slower and flow my speech. This helps me talk better.

CLINICIAN: Right! You know one way to help control your speech. What else have you learned?

STUTTERER: If I concentrate on moving my mouth and enunciate during speech, it makes the speech flow better.

CLINICIAN: Right again. How does all this make you feel about your speech?

STUTTERER: I'm more confident about being able to control my speech.

CLINICIAN: Your new, positive attitude is important to both your speech and your relations with other people. People enjoy being around you when you have a positive attitude. So, what happened? You said no one likes you.

STUTTERER: I guess I'm just feeling bad because I talked to someone and stuttered to them.

CLINICIAN: It's really good that you recognize it.

STUTTERER: But I couldn't control my speech with that person.

CLINICIAN: Did you stutter just as badly as you did when you started therapy?

STUTTERER: Well, no. It wasn't all that severe. But I still stuttered a little.

CLINICIAN: Then you did control your speech to some degree?

STUTTERER: I guess so. It wasn't as bad as it would have been before therapy.

CLINICIAN: Good thought! You are talking better.

STUTTERER: I guess I'll have to agree. My speech is better now than when I started therapy.

CLINICIAN: Very good! You recognize that you have made some progress.

In the above interaction, the clinician rewards the more positive coverants of the stutterer and penalizes the negative coverants. This approach could also be used on the aphasic as he makes statements to the effect that he can never fit into society again, that he is a burden to everyone, that he is helpless, that he will never get any better, and other such negative coverants. It can also be used with the client who has had a laryngectomy and is in a deep state of depression about his future. The clinician's rewards and penalties are used to modify the client's cognitive set by increasing the number of positive thoughts and decreasing the number of negative thoughts.

The Role of the CIM in Counseling

The CIM, being a communications model, is the core of all interactions in counseling. However, the clinician's tasks and responsibilities differ among the various counseling forms. In our discussion, we will concentrate on the variations in the clinician's stimulus, her cognitions, and her responses in the transaction.

There are both direct and indirect forms of cognitive counseling. In direct counseling, the clinician's stimulus is asking for information or suggesting answers to problems. In the indirect form, her stimulus is, for the most part, a reflection of the content (especially the feelings and emotions) of the client's responses. In some instances, she may ask the client to expand on something or, if the client is getting too far afield, ask a question that brings the client back to the topic. Her cognitions in both instances are concerned with evaluating the content of the client's communication. She is looking for cause-and-effect relationships and for cognitive distortions of reality. In direct cognitive counseling, this information assists in determining where the next transaction will go and what further questions need to be asked to clarify information already gathered. It also indicates when the clinician should provide some feedback to the client. In indirect cognitive counseling, the information gathered by the clinician tells the clinician where the counseling needs to be focused. The clinician's responses, in both forms, are noncommittal, neither agreeing nor disagreeing; they simply indicate that she is attending to the client. The changes in the cognitive set are accomplished through the client's own insights into the cognitive distortions.

In cognitive–behavioral counseling, the clinician's stimulus is behaviorally oriented, seeking clarification of interpretations of the behavioral performances or absence of the performances. The clinician is attempting to determine the client's reactions to his problematic behaviors. The clinician's cognitions are focused on attempting to determine if there is cognitive distortion involved in the perception of the behavior, such as seeing a defective behavior as normal or a normal behavior as defective. This information will determine where the next transaction will go. The clinician's responses here are the same as with cognitive counseling—simply supplying acknowledgments of what the client is saying. The cognitive set is changed through insights into the behavioral distortions.

The clinician's stimulus and cognitions in behavioral counseling are the same as with direct cognitive counseling or cognitive–behavioral counseling. The only difference lies in the clinician's responses. In this instance, the clinician provides responses that either reward positive thoughts or penalize negative thoughts. These rewards and penalties shape the cognitive set by influencing the frequency of positive and negative thoughts.

General Comments on Negative Cognitive Sets

Inventory of Assets and Liabilities

One of the best ways to see something objectively is to write it down. If you are feeling depressed, get a piece of paper and write down what is bothering you. You will be amazed at how quickly you can change your attitude once you examine the things that are bothering you. Things will not appear as foreboding once they are written down. We can use this technique with a client who has a negative cognitive set toward himself. I have my clients write out a detailed list of assets and liabilities. I tell them not to rush this, to take their time in completing the list. The longer they take, the shorter the list of liabilities (but they then include procrastination as a liability). When the list is finally completed, I go over it with the client and we talk about each item to see how valid it is. I often find that stuttering clients will take a characteristic such as sensitivity and put it in the column of liabilities. They insist that they are too sensitive to others' reactions. I do not argue this point, but I will point out that sensitivity to others' needs and feelings can be viewed as an asset.

Group Sharing

If you are providing group therapy for your clients, you have an opportunity to work on their emotional problems by allowing them to share their problems. Even though a client might have a problem in one area of his life, he might have some insights into problem areas of other clients. Group discussions of a particular client's problem provide the client with insights as to how others have dealt with similar problems. The clinician will need to monitor the group discussion and clarify points or suggest possible difficulties with proposed solutions. However, if the group members are all active in discussing each other's cognitive sets, all members of the group will profit from the experience. If the group is homogeneous, with all members having the same communicative disorder, the discussions are much more to the point and meaningful since members all share a common base. This type of group is especially good for stutterers, aphasics, and people with laryngectomies. I have found it advantageous at times to have the group consist of clients who are just entering therapy as well as clients who are well advanced in therapy. The more advanced clients can provide valuable insights for the beginning clients.

There is also the issue of credibility. A client is more apt to listen to a person who has resolved a similar problem than to a clinician who has never experienced the problem.

Referrals for Professional Counseling

To Supplement Speech Therapy

Consider the following situation. You are faced with clients whose emotional problems are such that you cannot deal with them, but they are interfering with your therapy. So you decide to make a referral for counseling as you continue with your therapy. This decision and procedure will most often be dictated by the agency where you are employed, but if you find yourself in such a situation and have a choice in terms of the referral, I have some suggestions to make. The most important criterion in this instance is to find a psychologist or psychiatrist who will work *with* you. You must coordinate your therapy with the counseling the client is receiving. This calls for good communication between you and the counselor, which is not always easy. I have found it wise to have a meeting with the psychologist or psychiatrist to discuss coordinating the treatment programs. One sure sign of a bad choice for a referral is if the counselor will not take the time to have a conference with you. I have also found it very important that the psychologist or psychiatrist appreciate the role of my profession and respect me as a professional. If I do not get this, I know I will not be able to coordinate the treatment programs.

When you decide that you want to refer a client for counseling, consider the orientation of the person to whom you might refer your client. You will find, generally, two basic orientations for treatment. One is cognitive, which we discussed earlier in this chapter. The second orientation is psychoanalytic, based on Freudian concepts. The most typical psychoanalytic approach is indirect, following the guidelines presented earlier. The two treatment methods are vastly different, and therefore, you may want to get some consultation on this matter before you make your referral.

The other choice you have is between a psychologist and a psychiatrist, both of whom specialize in the study of the human mind and its functions. The psychologist is not medically oriented and cannot prescribe medication. He or she has majored in psychology for many years and has either a master's degree or a doctoral degree. A psychologist's orientation is almost always cognitive.

A psychiatrist is a physician who specializes in psychology. He or she can prescribe medication and often includes this as part of a treatment program.

Many psychiatrists work purely under the medical model, while others have a psychodynamic (cognitive) or a Freudian psychoanalytic orientation.

In Place of Speech Therapy

Situations also occur where you will decide that the client needs professional counseling before he is ready for speech therapy. With this type of client, there are so many emotional problems in his life that he cannot effectively deal with your treatment. Perhaps you attempted to work with the client, but your therapy did not produce the desired effects. The client behaves in bizarre ways, and most of your attempts at therapy are out of your control. I have seen a lot of speech therapy like this, even when the client has no emotional problems. We discussed this earlier as awful therapy. If you find yourself in a situation like this, where the client's emotional problems prevent your working with him, it is time to make a referral. It is not as important here to find a professional who will communicate with you, since you are not attempting to coordinate two treatment programs. But it is wise to make sure that there is some communication so you know when you should reintroduce your treatment program. Again, this must be coordinated through your agency and the client's family. Your actions depend on the policy of the agency where you work.

Negative Cognitive Sets in Significant Others

Significant others often interfere with therapy with their negative attitudes and responses to the client's particular communication disorder. In previous chapters, we have discussed shifting their role from an S− to an S+ or an S0 by changing their response from a penalty to a reward or at least to a neutral response. In most cases, a negative response on the part of the significant others is not meant to be disruptive; it is a response that comes naturally from frustration, or from not understanding the nature of the client's problem. We can assist the significant others most effectively by providing them with information about the client's disorder. We can also tell them how to respond. For example, the parents of a child who stutters may respond to their child's stuttering by becoming frustrated and angry because they do not understand why the child cannot say the word properly. They constantly yell at the child to stop stuttering. When the parents understand the nature of stuttering and that the child really wants to say the word but cannot, they will more than likely be able to change their response. We could even tell them to be patient with the child and give him time to get the words out. Significant others are not out to destroy your therapy, they are just human.

However, there are some significant others who may purposely work against your therapy because of their own needs. They may be so emotionally involved with the client and his disorder that they respond rather irrationally. I was once working with a 6-year-old, severely involved cerebral palsied girl, and part of my treatment consisted of teaching her to feed herself. I would make very good progress during each therapy session, but when the child returned for the following session, she had lost everything I had taught her two days earlier. This had gone on for about 2 weeks when the social worker in the agency called me in for a conference on the child. She had been working with the mother on her emotional involvement with the child. The mother had a great deal of guilt associated with giving birth to a severely disabled child. She compensated for her guilt by waiting on the child constantly. She would even get up every hour during the night and turn the child over. The child became her "crown of thorns," her source of punishment for what she had done.

As the child became more independent and did not need her help as much, the mother felt she was losing her crown of thorns, which she needed in order to deal with her guilt. One of the things she was doing in order to maintain the child's dependence on her was to slap the child's hands if she attempted to feed herself. I then understood why I could not achieve progress with the child. The mother had established herself as an S− for self-feeding behaviors. Obviously, this situation could not be corrected by giving the mother information about the disorder. The mother needed professional help in dealing with her emotional problems associated with her handicapped child.

Although this type of situation may be the exception rather then the rule, these clinical situations do exist and must be dealt with in a most professional manner. If you do not have a social worker or psychologist in your agency to turn to, you might contact the family physician and seek his advice. Just be certain you operate within the rules of the agency where you are working. In this type of situation, the significant other needs as much help as the client.

Finally, there are those significant others who are undermining your therapy due to some personal factor unknown to you. You find you are making no progress because of the significant others' responses, and you have no way of changing their attitudes or responses. They reject even the most subtle reference to counseling. What do you do here? This depends again on your agency's procedures. If you have a waiting list of clients who would profit from your therapy, you must consider how to make the most effective and efficient use of your clinical time. You may have to dismiss the client, as regrettable as this may be, so another client can profit from therapy. I once worked with a young boy who stuttered and was making very significant progress when the father suddenly removed him from therapy. I discussed this with the father, but his only response was that his child would just have to learn to live with it and "be a man." He justified his yelling at the child by explaining that it "toughened him up." No amount of discussion could change the father's attitude. This is a situation you just must accept, regardless of the moral and ethical issues involved. Child abuse takes many forms.

CLINICAL SUPERVISION: AN OVERVIEW

◆ Synopsis

Supervision of therapy is an essential ingredient if the clinician's clinical skills are to improve. Supervision is defined and clinical teaching is discussed as part of this chapter. The chapter's philosophical tone is tempered by a practical view of the interaction between the supervisor and the clinician, the Supervision Clinical Interaction Model (SCIM). The role of the SCIM in supervision is discussed as part of the clinician's learning experience.

Clinical supervision is basically evaluation of therapy, and it is a learning process for both the clinician and the supervisor. The clinician has now put together all her knowledge and insights into an ongoing, interpersonal learning interaction with a client (i.e., therapy), and the supervisor is observing it and evaluating how well it is functioning. The teaching/learning occurs during the conference the supervisor has with the clinician. The supervisor learns as she integrates what she has observed with her own clinical experiences and attempts to explain this to the clinician. The clinician learns by seeing her therapy from a different perspective—that of a skilled and objective professional.

Rather than write a chapter dealing with the underlying theories and practices of supervision, I chose to edit various materials from the *Handbook of Supervision: A Cognitive Behavioral System* (Leith, McNiece, & Fusilier, 1989). When I reviewed the book in preparation for writing this chapter, I found that not only did the materials cover what I wanted to say, but it was so well written that I did not feel I could improve on it. Adapted information from that book follows.

Clinical Supervision: A Definition

We must start our discussion by attempting to define the term "supervision." Perhaps if we break it down logically into two words, "super" and "vision," it will give us some indication of what supervision is. The term "super" means either "extraordinary" or "over something." Then we consider the second word, "vision." This is defined as the act or power of sight or seeing. The first combination of definitions that comes into focus would imply that supervision is "extraordinary sight." If this is hindsight, this is not too bad a definition of supervision since, at least in my experience, the supervisory conference considers mistakes that have already been made. However, if it is foresight, we are in trouble, since it would seem to suggest that we should "foresee" all clinical problems and avoid them. Clearly, this perfect therapy is out of the range of most clinicians and even supervisors.

The second combination of definitions, "extraordinary seeing," would seem to refer to someone who has exceptional eyesight. In thinking this over, a large number of the supervisors I have known wore eyeglasses. This would seem to exclude them from having exceptional eyesight. In fact, some of them did not even have exceptional insight or hindsight.

The third combination, "over sight," seems to refer to the clinical mistakes that clinicians make, rather than being descriptive of supervision. In fact, "over sight" seems to be more the reason supervision is needed than a definition of it. Perhaps oversight is the justification for supervision.

Our last combination is "over seeing," and since it is the last combination, it had better be a good one. Supervision or clinical supervision, according to this definition, means that the clinical interactions between the clinician and the client are being overseen by someone. We can then further imply that the person who is overseeing the clinical work is called a "clinical supervisor," and that he or she has expertise in the particular interaction. If there is no expertise, then the person is not overseeing but rather simply observing, which I will discuss shortly.

Good supervision is a skill that is learned over time. To dispel a common misunderstanding, supervisory skill is not correlated with academic accomplishment. Just because an individual has achieved a doctorate does not mean that he or she is a qualified supervisor. They might be able to perform in an indirect supervisory mode, where they act as a resource and can call on their knowledge of the literature. However, in direct supervision, where the supervisor is evaluating clinical performance, the criterion for a good supervisor is experience as a clinician, regardless of academic degrees. Supervisors cannot evaluate and judge a process that they are not totally familiar with, no matter the amount of their knowledge of information or literature about any particular disorder. This means that a supervisor must be able to call upon her many years of experience as a clinician in her evaluation of clinical performances. It also means that the supervisor should have been an outstanding clinician during her clinical years. I do not mean to imply that all good clinicians automatically are good supervisors. As I said earlier, supervisory skills are learned. The supervisor must know what she is looking for when she observes therapy. She must have the tools to describe what is happening in therapy and communicate this while suggesting changes in the clinical process to the clinician. She needs to be able to lead the clinician toward solving her clinical problems. Special training is necessary to learn these skills. Unfortunately, the amount and kind of training necessary to achieve this level of supervisory skill has yet to be determined; much investigation is still needed in this area.

Evaluation

We cannot leave this discussion without considering the term *evaluation* as it relates to supervision. Evaluation is part of supervision. It is through the supervisory process that the supervisor is able to evaluate the clinical performance of a clinician. This is the part of the supervisory process that yields the clinical grade for the clinician still in training. And it is this part of the supervisory process that is usually the most subjective and, in many cases, vague and ambiguous. The clinician wants to know what behaviors or actions she is being judged on and what the criteria are for grading; here, most clinical supervisory procedures break down, since there are no standard, operational definitions of the clinical behaviors being observed and evaluated (see Appendix B). Further, there are no specific criteria for grading performance. This is the basis for the anxiety found in many clinicians involved in supervised clinical experiences.

Observation

We also need to consider the differences between supervision and observation. Although observation may be a part of supervision, supervision is not necessarily a part of observation. Anyone can observe something—all it takes is watching. There are observation ports in the barriers at many construction sites so people can watch the construction. These people, fortunately, are only observing, not supervising, the construction. Observation is a popular activity at beaches. Men are observing women in their bathing suits at the same time women are observing men in their bathing suits. This is called observers observing observers. And we all recognize that there is no supervision involved in the observation of people at the beach. A lot of judgments and ratings perhaps, but no supervision.

And, let us not forget, each of us started out in the profession by observing clinicians, usually other students about a year ahead of us, doing therapy. We were deeply engrossed in observing the clinical interactions, wondering why the clinician was doing certain things and wondering how the clinician would react to specific things the client did in therapy. Little did we know that the clinician was wondering the same things at the same time. Our clinical observations were a learning experience for us. They gave us some insight into what the profession was all about. But, and I am certain you will agree, you were not in a position at that time to supervise the clinician.

The overseer or supervisor must have special knowledge and expertise in order to supervise. Therefore, the supervisor is an expert, knowledgeable of all aspects of the event he or she is supervising. And the supervisor's observations are the basis for his or her professional appraisal of the quality and quantity of the thing they are supervising.

Observation for clinical assessment is a unique form of observation. Anderson (1988) writes "Observation to some *is* supervision." She goes on to say that in the literature on supervision, the terms "*observation* and *supervision* are often used interchangeably." Perhaps the problem with some clinical supervisors is that they do not understand the distinct difference between *observation* and *supervision*. This invaluable clinical skill must be clearly developed, and is not automatically acquired through clinical experience.

The Learning Experience: Hindsight, Insight, Foresight

How many times have you heard someone say that clinical supervision is a learning experience? Well, until there is a supervisory meeting between the clinician who did the therapy and the supervisor who observed the clinical interactions, the supervision is usually a learning experience only for the supervisor. She may never have seen therapy done that way before, and she may hope she never sees it done that way again.

Once there is a meeting between the supervisor and the clinician, the conference can be a learning experience for the clinician as well. The type of interaction between the clinician and the supervisor will determine if learn-ing takes place. The most basic ingredient needed in this interaction is good communication that includes well-defined topics, a commonly understood vocabulary, commonly understood concepts, and an active interchange of knowledge between the supervisor and the clinician. If there is not good communication, learning is severely impaired.

The purpose of the clinical supervision meeting is for the clinician to gain insight into her interactions with her client. She needs to know what she did wrong in the interaction and why it was wrong. She also needs to appreciate what she did correctly and why her action was correct. The end result of the conference should be that the clinician has a deeper and broader understanding of what transpired in the therapy session. And from this better understanding of the clinical interactions, there should be better therapy planning for future clinical sessions and some foresight so that incorrect behaviors do not occur again.

Now, let us see if I can put this all together in a simple statement. If I failed to do this, it would be an oversight on my part, or perhaps I would be short-sighted. So I will say that clinical hindsight is the base of clinical insight, which in turn provides us with clinical foresight that is the base of good therapy. Or, put another way, hindsight leads to insight which gives us foresight. Why don't you stop here for a second and reread the last two sentences to make sure you have it.

Clinical Teaching

In this discussion of teaching, let us consider the clinician's role in therapy. I feel her purpose in therapy is to teach the client new speech or language behaviors, new concepts, new thoughts, and so forth. This is clinical teaching. The beginning clinician must learn various teaching methods to use with her clients. It is assumed that she learns to teach by using modeling—giving the client guidance in behavioral performance, using rewards and penalties—or through the cognitive process by providing the client with information about a behavior performance, concept, or belief. However, it must then be asked, who is teaching the new clinician how to teach? The first step in learning appears to be through observation; that is, watching another clinician doing therapy and then trying to imitate the model. Unfortunately, as was just pointed out, the other clinician being observed is usually another student clinician who is just as confused as the observer. This is somewhat akin to trying to learn to swim by watching someone drown. However, right or wrong, the foundations of therapy interactions are established here. They must then be modified, shaped if you please, into a professional approach to therapy and clinical interaction. This, then, is the role of the supervisor, the clinical teacher.

Clinical teaching is a term often used to imply that there are two distinct areas of teaching: academic teaching and clinical teaching. Ask any clinician where they learned to do therapy and they will tell you they learned it, not in their regular academic courses, but in a special school, the school of hard knocks. They had to become involved in the therapy interaction before they could learn the intricacies of the clinical process. And they needed to be guided through the process by an experienced clinician who would observe their therapy and discuss it with them. This person was their clinical supervisor, their clinical teacher. This teacher, as with all teachers, used various teaching methods, ranging from direct teaching (in the form of a lecture that passed information to the clinician) to indirect teaching (in the form of discussions and providing references for the clinician to help resolve clinical problems). The former method seems more appropriate for beginning clinicians, while the latter would be used with the advanced clinician.

Another way to look at clinical teaching is that the supervisor is primarily concerned with *how* the client is being taught, while the academic teacher is more concerned with *what* the client is being taught. This is not to say that there is no overlap between the teachers, only that each has a particular focus. The supervisor's focus is on therapy while the academic teacher is more concerned with providing information about a particular disorder so the student can plan an appropriate treatment program.

Continuing this one step further, most academic courses are disorder-oriented; they are concerned with presenting the student with information about a particular disorder. The student is presented with information concerning the etiology, behavioral descriptions, emotional aspects, and basic research into the disorder. On the other hand, clinical teaching, direct or indirect, is more global in scope. It is not limited specifically to a disorder, but rather to the disorder as it relates to a particular client. It involves discussions and/or lectures, depending on the orientation of the supervisor, concerning interactional transactions, client motivation and attention, and teaching strategies. To put it more succinctly, academic teaching is more concerned with the theoretical aspects of disorders while clinical teaching is concerned with the pragmatics of therapy or treatment. Both areas of teaching must be present for the complete training of the clinician. Many supervisors incorporate both of these areas of teaching into their supervision.

Supervisory Transactions

Earlier, we established the clinician/client interactions as being a series of transactions based on a stimulus–organism–response (S–O–R) exchange. The concept of the clinical transaction was developed into a model, the CIM. Because interactions between the supervisor and the clinician are also based on this S–O–R exchange, only minor modifications are necessary to make the original transaction model applicable to supervision. It is only necessary to change the two participants in the transactions, replacing "clinician" with "supervisor" and "client" with "clinician." Thus, the first half of the transaction, S–O–R, represents the supervisor presenting the stimulus (S) to the clinician, the organism (O) for cognition. The clinician then provides the response (R), and the first half of the transaction is complete.

The second half of the transaction, S–O–R/S–O–R, represents the response of the clinician in becoming the stimulus (S) for the supervisor who, as the organism (O), cognates the response and then responds (R) to the clinician. This interaction constitutes one transaction. The next transaction builds on the results of this transaction. Each transaction is again dependent upon the previous transaction.

In the clinical conference, each transaction constitutes a transfer of information, with the supervisor giving information to the clinician or requesting information from her. The supervisor must determine basically if the information she sent was received properly and if the information she requested is correct. So each transaction is tested by the supervisor after the clinician has responded.

The clinician's response, even when she asks questions, provides the supervisor with insight into the status of the information that is being exchanged in the clinical conference. The supervisor needs to determine from the clinician's response the correctness of the response, the depth and thoroughness of the response, the problem-solving process the clinician used, and what the stimulus should be to start the next transaction. If the transaction has been successful, the supervisor rewards the clinician and then moves ahead in the transactional process. However, if the transaction has not been successful—the clinician did not learn properly—the supervisor responds with a slight penalty, such as saying, "That's not quite right. Let me explain that again." She then repeats the transaction, making a correction in her stimulus so it is more appropriate for the academic and clinical level of the clinician.

The Role of the SCIM
in the Supervision Conference

In Chapter 3, the Clinical Interaction Model (CIM) was developed to illustrate the detailed interactions between the clinician and the client. We now modify the model to the Supervisory Clinical Interaction Model (SCIM) so that it applies to the interactions between the clinician and the supervisor (see Figure 12.1). Let us discuss the changes according to the supervisor's stimulus, cognitions, and response during the interaction.

The Supervisor's Stimulus (S)

The supervisor's stimulus is made up of modeling, guidance, and information. The most important of the teaching strategies for the supervisor is giving information to and requesting information from the clinician. She provides the clinician with information about such things as her clinical plan, her clinical performance, the type of client she is working with, her problem-solving strategies, and so forth. She also requests information from the clinician to assess her retention of information, the process of information recall, and the process used for problem solving. The focal point of the clinical conference is the exchange of information and the assessment of the clinician's cognitions.

The Clinician's Cognitions and Response (O–R–/S)

The cognitive activity the clinician engages in during any given transaction is dependent upon the supervisor's stimulus. If the supervisor is giving the clinician information, the clinician is thinking about information being presented, attempting to commit it to memory, and trying to associate it with some relevant clinical factor, such as the client she is working with, the type of test she is performing, and so forth. The cognitive function here is one of committing to memory as much information as possible.

This is also a "sorting and stacking" activity, where information is put into categories for storage and easy retrieval. No response is required here, as long as the supervisor continues to give information or until she requests one. If the supervisor shifts her approach and, instead of providing information,

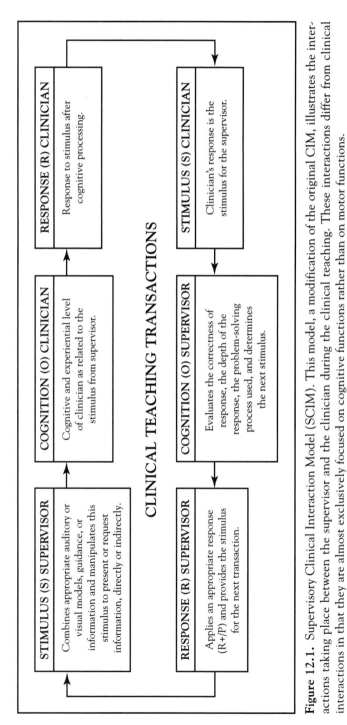

Figure 12.1. Supervisory Clinical Interaction Model (SCIM). This model, a modification of the original CIM, illustrates the interactions taking place between the supervisor and the clinician during the clinical teaching. These interactions differ from clinical interactions in that they are almost exclusively focused on cognitive functions rather than on motor functions.

requests information, the cognitive activity of the clinician must shift from information storage to information retrieval. In order to respond to the questions asked by the supervisor, the clinician must draw upon both her long- and short-term memory.

The clinician has three basic responses to the supervisor, which depend on the cognitive activity taking place in the conference. If the supervisor is providing information and then asking specific questions about what was said, such as, "What muscles are involved in this action?" The clinician is expected to respond to the question. The second response type is for the clinician to answer a question that the supervisor directs to her, but that is not directly related to information that has just been presented. The third response form, which might appear to be spontaneous but is really prompted directly or indirectly by the supervisor, involves the clinician asking the supervisor questions.

The clinician's response, whatever it is, becomes the stimulus for the supervisor. This is what she responds to. It is the clinician's response that the supervisor analyzes to determine the focus of the next clinical transaction.

The Supervisor's Cognitions (O)

The first cognition the supervisor must perform is to estimate the cognitive knowledge level of the clinician. This cognitive level is related to the clinician's academic and clinical knowledge, and it establishes the stimulus level the supervisor will provide. This estimate may indeed be incorrect, either too high or too low, but the supervisor must establish a starting point. She may revise the estimate as she explores the clinician's cognitions in each clinical transaction.

Each transaction must be tested before the next transaction can commence. The supervisor must determine if the transaction was successfully completed before she can move ahead in whatever activity she is engaged. The type of testing the supervisor does depends on the purpose of the transaction. For example, if the transaction is for providing the clinician with some information, the supervisor must determine if the information was received correctly before proceeding to the next bit of information.

In another mode, the supervisor asks the clinician to resolve a hypothetical clinical problem. She gives the clinician the necessary information about the situation, and then asks, "As you know, the client has a severe hearing loss and, due to cerebral palsy, also has problems with fine motor movements. How would you approach teaching this client to produce the [s] sound?" The clinician is now called upon to utilize her academic and clinical knowledge (and her sorting and stacking) to solve the clinical problem. Her response will be the result of her cognitive evaluation of the problem and its apparent solution. The supervisor is now evaluating the correctness of the response.

The final cognitive mode has to do with responding to questions asked by the clinician. After inviting and receiving questions, the supervisor must not only think of appropriate answers but also evaluate the quality of the questions themselves. She must determine if the questions reflect a severe lack of knowledge or confusion in the area, or if this is just a minor point that can be cleared up by answering the question. She also needs to be aware of why the questions are being asked. Is this a true search for answers to questions or a ploy to gain attention, distract from other issues, or try to impress her?

The Supervisor's Response (R)

It is extremely important for the supervisor to respond to the clinician at the end of each transaction. Rewards for the clinician should be of a social nature—actions or words on the part of the supervisor that convey approval. The challenge for the supervisor is to come up with forms of approval that are clear to the clinician and that do not fade to the point that they are meaningless.

Even though most supervisors deny using penalty as a teaching tool, it is an integral part of almost every supervisory conference. Penalty may take the form of a frown on the supervisor's face, as the clinician is presenting her solution to a clinical problem. Or it may be the supervisor saying, "Well, that's not quite right." Some people call this negative feedback, but it is just penalty packaged under a different label. Penalty is anything that the clinician finds even slightly aversive, and it is a very powerful teaching tool. When used in conjunction with reward, the combination is almost unbeatable.

Self-Supervision

All clinicians need to continue the supervisory process if they are going to continue to develop their clinical skills. The solution to continuing development is "self-supervision." Self-supervision is the ability of the clinician not only to recognize clinical problems when they arise in therapy, but to solve the problems. First, the clinician must be sensitive to problems that arise and impede the efficiency or effectiveness of her therapy. This awareness of clinical problems must be present at all times. The clinician cannot allow a problem to exist for several months and then suddenly recognize it. She must be constantly assessing her therapy. It is only after she becomes aware of problems that she can attempt to solve them. She must consider all the factors operating in the clinical interactions and, by carefully examining all the factors, determine if a relationship exists between them and the clinical problem she is facing. If she discovers a corresponding relationship, she will therefore discover how to deal with it. If the clinician cannot recognize her clinical problems and resolve them in an orderly and logical way, she will never be able to function effectively as a professional clinician.

The following is from the preface of this book:

> Therapy is not a mystical procedure. It is a learning situation that is based on learning principles that govern the interaction between the clinician and the client. Once the principles are understood, therapeutic interaction becomes a lawful process that can be planned, and its outcome can be predicted.

I now add this: Since it is a lawful interaction, it can be supervised by anyone who understands the principles, including the clinician herself.

CHAPTER

THE PHENOMENON OF STUTTERING

◆ Synopsis

Of all the communication disorders, the most baffling is stuttering. It fits no particular pattern or style for the individual stutterer; it is inconsistent as to the severity of each stutterer's speech in various situations; it is much more prevalent in males than in females; once stuttering is established, there is no known cure for the stuttering; many children eventually outgrow stuttering and speak normally the remainder of their lives; stuttering usually begins between the ages of 3 and 5, but there are cases where stuttering begins in the late teens; and the list of incongruities continues. The disorder of stuttering is a conundrum in the fields of speech pathology and psychology.

This book focuses on clinical methods. The clinical methods are based on the principles of cognitive–behavioral therapy. A review of the literature reveals only one cognitive–behavioral therapy program for stuttering and that book is out of print. A synopsis of the cognitive–behavioral stuttering therapy program from that book is presented here. It includes both the cognitive and the behavioral aspects, as well as therapy techniques to minimize stuttering and terminate stuttering blocks should they occur. The therapy programs are presented for both adults and children who stutter.

The Challenge

Why does this chapter on cognitive–behavioral therapy for stuttering appear in a book on general clinical methods in speech pathology? Well, the general clinical methods are also based on cognitive–behavioral therapy. When I checked the literature, there was only one cognitive–behavioral treatment plan offered for stuttering (Leith, 1984), and that book is out of print. So, in order to relate my book on clinical methods to stuttering therapy, the chapter needed to be here. And, it is time to renew the profession's acquaintance with the therapy program because it has been unavailable for several years. Plus I think, after using the plan myself for almost 20 years, that it is a very effective and efficient therapy program.

Stuttering is a distinctive communication disorder. It shares nothing with any other communication disorder in etiology, speech manifestations, emotional involvement, associated behaviors, or any other factor. We feel that stuttering should be considered an independent disorder type, as are language disorders, rather than being conjoined with articulation and voice disorders.

For many years, the speech pathologist has been trained in stuttering therapy along the lines of a behavior orientation (Ingham, 1984) or a cognitive orientation (Van Riper, 1973). We are suggesting cognitive–behavioral therapy orientation (Meichenbaum, 1977), which is distinctly different from either a behavioral therapy orientation or a cognitive therapy orientation. Although the distinction between cognitive–behavioral therapy and behavior therapy has not caused any confusion among psychologists, the same cannot be said of cognitive–behavioral therapy and cognitive therapy. Radnitz (2000) states that the terms *cognitive–behavioral therapy* and *cognitive therapy* are often used interchangeably professionally. Further, Dobson and Block (1988) state that cognitive–behavioral therapies share three basic assumptions. First, that cognitions can affect behaviors. Second, that cognitions can be identified and changed. And third, that alteration in thinking can lead to positive changes in behavior. Additionally, according to Beck (1976), cognitive therapy is often considered only a subset of cognitive–behavioral therapy. We shall conclude that cognitive–behavioral therapy is an entity within itself, separate from behavior therapy, but closely allied with cognitive therapy.

The remainder of the chapter will be focused on the cognitive–behavioral therapy approach to stuttering. We will discuss the behaviors and cognitions associated with stuttering, how the stuttering starts, where it occurs, and techniques to minimize stuttering when it occurs and to terminate the stuttering episodes. We will present treatment for both the adult and the child who stutter.

The Rationale

The professional charge of the speech pathologist was, at one time, to provide treatment for those disorders related to communication—disorders of articulation, voice, stuttering, and language. However, when the list of disorders was carefully examined, it was seen that one disorder was obviously of a different genre—language disorders. In recognizing this difference, the professional organization was renamed the American Speech-Language-Hearing Association. Hence, the speech pathologist is now charged with treating the speech disorders of articulation, voice, and stuttering, along with some unique disorders such as a swallowing disorder, which has an organic etiology, and spasmodic dysphonia, which has a vague, undetermined etiology.

If we look carefully at this arrangement, we are once again faced with the problem of mixed genres. This time, though, the problem is not as straightforward as the original one involving language disorders. This one involves several problems of incompatibility between stuttering on one hand and articulation and voice disorders on the other.

The most troubling factor is with the consistency of error of the disorders. Articulation errors are found in the production of specific phonemes. Errors involve substitution of one sound for another, the omission of a needed sound in a word, the distortion of a particular sound, and the addition of an unwanted sound to a word. These errors range from faulty learning of the sound to physiological factors, such as paralysis or hearing loss.

Voice disorders are usually related to the physiology of vocal production. Vocal pitch may be too high or too low, or problems may be related to the uncontrolled variability of pitch. Vocal volume may be too loud or too soft or related to the uncontrolled variability of loudness. Voice quality is a bit more complex reflecting a whole range of descriptions: hoarse, harsh, metallic, strident, tinny, muffled, and many other terms describing the deviant voice quality. Again, this involves a horse of a different color; all of these conditions are related to the physiological make up of the larynx.

There are several areas of conflict we must deal with when attempting to consider these disorders as a single unit, a single grouping of "speech disorders," as opposed to "language disorders." Although these disorders do incorporate the same physiological factors (breathing, phonation, and articulation), they are separated into two distinct categories when considering the consistency of their communication errors. Both articulation and voice disorders have strong error consistency in their clients. If a client produces a sound incorrectly, the error occurs whenever the suspect sound is produced in the phonetic error position in the speech. Also, if a client has a voice disorder, the phonology error in production occurs whenever the client phonates. Both are error consistent; the clients systematically produce the error as they articulate or phonate, except, we hope, after therapy. However, the client who stutters differs drastically in this respect.

The client who stutters has wide variations in frequency of stuttering, i.e., from being totally free of stuttering in some speaking situations to experiencing severe stuttering in others. This is related to the stress or anxiety the client encounters in the speaking situation. If he is speaking to a child, talking to a dog, or speaking alone in an open field, he will more than likely be completely fluent. A wide variation in severity is a common occurrence with all stutterers.

In the same vein, all stutterers have periods of time when, regardless of stress, they speak completely fluently, be it for a short period of time, measured in minutes, or for an extended time, measured in months. This event is not dependent on any therapy on the stutterer's part; it occurs spontaneously. However, it ends just as unexpectedly, and the stutterer resumes his stuttering at the same severity level as previously experienced. It goes without saying that this event, the failure of fluency, is emotionally disturbing for the stutterer who was led to believe, even for a short period of time, that he was cured of his stuttering.

Still another factor that sets aside the two groups of disorders is that of client emotional involvement in the disorder. If, indeed, the client with an articulation/voice disorder has an emotional problem, it is highly unlikely that the emotional problem is directly related to the speech disorder. To the speech pathologist, emotional issues are not a common etiological factor in either articulation disorders or voice disorders, although they may be indirectly related.

The stutterer is directly and irrevocably tied to the emotional problems related to stuttering. As the stuttering develops, from about 3 to 5 years of age, the child becomes aware of his helplessness to correct or control the stuttering. He attempts to rid himself of the stuttering by modifying his speech, adopting both verbal mannerisms and nonverbal behaviors that are foreign to him, attempting to "force" sounds out, blinking his eyes, grimacing, and so forth. He gradually learns he is helpless to change the behaviors, hence the term "learned helplessness" coined by professional writers in psychology (Garber & Seligman, 1980; Seligman, 1975). At this point, he is changing to a confirmed, or secondary, stutterer. He continues to adopt secondary mannerisms, attempting to avoid stuttering or force words out until early adulthood, where he settles on a repertoire of mannerisms in his attempts to control his stuttering. In all likelihood, fear, frustration, anxiety, anger, and avoidance have by this time become an integral part of the paradigm of stuttering.

So even when an individual is considered a confirmed stutterer, he will still have periods of false fluency and will experience total fluency in some select speaking situations. When you add this factor to the emotional aspects of stuttering, it is obvious that the speech defects of articulation and voice disorders are different from the problems faced in stuttering.

We must also consider that there are other forms of stuttering that fit into the paradigm. Stuttering is loosely defined as speech where repetitions and/or prolongations of sounds, syllables, or articulatory positions, voiced or unvoiced, interrupt the forward flow of speech.

This very general operational definition not only fits the most common form of stuttering, developmental stuttering; it also fits the "hysterical," or "psychogenic," form of psychological stuttering (Culatta & Goldberg, 1995; Manning, 2001) and the "organic," or "neurogenic," stuttering (Culatta & Goldberg, 1995; Manning, 2001) that is associated with neurological insult. However, the latter two classifications represent a completely unique form of stuttering—a major departure from the classical form represented in the developmental variety of stuttering.

One the most baffling aspects of the psychogenic form of stuttering is the presence of La Belle Indifference, wherein the client is oblivious to the fact that he or she is stuttering severely. It is even more incredulous when you consider the form the stuttering takes: very rapid and lengthy repetitions on almost every word spoken. Clients speak with no emotional reaction to the severe interruptions in the flow of their speech. Typically, these stutterers demonstrate extremely rapid and rhythmic repetitions and a lack of emotion or struggle during the extended disruption of the flow of speech. Treatment of these clients involves special strategies and techniques, most of which are foreign to the typical speech pathologist.

One final form of a purely rhythmic disorder is listed in many references as "cluttering" (Manning, 2001; St. Louis & Myers, 1997). In clutterring, the client speaks at such a rapid rate he "stumbles over his words." This is not classified as a form of stuttering and, in its pure form, is quite rare. Used car salesmen and other fast-talkers do not fit in the label of cluttering.

Before starting our chapter on stuttering therapy, I ask you to review the materials in Chapters 3 and 4. The material covered in those pages is basic to the cognitive–behavioral stuttering therapy which will be presented in this chapter. Pay particular attention to the sections on the Clinical Interaction Model (CIM), stimulus manipulation, and conditioned stimuli.

A Cognitive–Behavioral Approach to Stuttering Therapy

A review of the literature reveals only one therapy reference based on cognitive–behavioral therapy (Leith, 1984). Although that book is now out of print, a summary of that work was combined with a second article on cognitive–behavioral therapy (Leith, 2000) to form the final chapter in this book.

Impairment, Disability, or a Handicap

Which term should be used to describe a person who stutters? Is he impaired, does he have a disability, or is he handicapped? The World Health Organization (WHO, 1980) addressed this issue and created a model for general handicapping conditions. Yaruss (1998) expanded the original WHO model specifically for stuttering. Yaruss' model includes three levels of speech impairment, speech disability, and speech handicaps. These are listed below, each followed by a short descriptive comment: impairment of speech fluency (blocking); impairment of emotion, affect, or mood (anxiety); and impairment of behavioral pattern (avoidance). Disability includes disability of talking (limited verbal output); disability in work performance (talking at work); and situation coping disability (inability to perform specifics). Handicap includes occupational handicap (failure in occupation); social handicap (failure socially); and economic handicap (failure to achieve).

We start our discussion of stuttering by considering the behavioral aspects, because it is the stuttering behavior itself that is the basis of the negative cognitive set or mental attitude of the stutterer. Once we have considered the behaviors associated with stuttering, we can better understand the stutterer's cognitive reaction to the phenomenon.

Behavioral Aspects of Stuttering

The Stuttering Block. First, let us examine an operational description of stuttering. We can work from this base as we examine the behavioral events that constitute what we refer to as stuttering. The disorder of stuttering is not a single behavioral event, but rather is made up of a combination of interrelated behaviors.

Stuttering consists of repetitions and/or prolongations of sounds, syllables, and words. Furthermore, all individuals who stutter have, in varying degrees, both repetitions and/or prolongations in their speech. These repetitions and/or prolongations vary according to the frequency of occurrence in the speech (e.g. one occurrence in every 10 words), the intensity of their occurrence (e.g., each occurrence associated with severe struggle behavior), and the duration of their occurrence (e.g., each occurrence lasting 1 second). This then constitutes the block, the interruption of the forward moving flow of speech. The phenomenon is even more complex when you consider other behavioral aspects of stuttering. So, we will consider the repetitions and prolongations as follows:

- *Repetition.* The repetition is an inappropriate repeating of an articulatory position or movement that impedes the forward movement of speech.

- *Prolongations.* The prolongation is an inappropriate prolonging of an articulatory position that impedes the forward movement of speech.

Secondary Mannerisms. In addition to the repetitions and prolongations, there are other behaviors that the individual uses to avoid or terminate the repetitions and prolongations by diverting the client's attention from his stuttering blocks. These behaviors are referred to as secondary mannerisms, accessory features, or anxiety-reducing behaviors. They occur in an attempt by the stutterer to avoid or terminate a repetition or prolongation. They are a manifestation of the fear, anxiety, and frustration the client has regarding his stuttering. The mannerism, as such, never occurs unless it is associated with a stuttering block, either in anticipation of a block or during a block itself. Mannerisms are divided into *verbal mannerisms*, which are directly related to the speech, and *nonverbal mannerisms*, which are related to bodily movements.

Verbal Mannerisms. The verbal mannerisms, behaviors that are directly related to the speech, would include the following:

- *Language modifiers.* Sounds, words, or phrases the stutterer uses to avoid or terminate the block are referred to as language modifiers.

- *Retrials.* Words or phrases repeated inappropriately to avoid or terminate stuttering.

- *Rate of speech.* An inappropriately rapid rate of speech is used to avoid stuttering, i.e., to get the words out before the stuttering occurs.

- *Postponement.* Occurs when the stutterer postpones his speech and remains silent until he feels he can speak without stuttering.

Nonverbal Mannerisms. These behavioral mannerisms are not directly related to the speech. They are general motor movements that occur and distract the stutterer.

- *Eye gestures.* The term *eye gestures* includes eye blinks, eye closures, eye movements, eye contact, or any other mannerism involving the eyes that the stutterer uses to avoid or terminate the stuttering block.

- *Tongue movements.* Tongue movements include such things as tongue protrusion, tongue clicks or smacks, or other such inappropriate tongue movements used to avoid or terminate the block.

- *Mouth movements.* Pursing of the lips, opening the mouth very wide, and other such inappropriate mouth movements are included in this classification.

- *Head movements.* When the head is nodded, jerked upward or downward, or turned in any direction in order to influence the stuttering, the movement is a nonverbal mannerism.

- *Body movements.* Nonverbal mannerisms in this category include such things as arm movement swings, foot movements, finger or foot tapping, or gross body movements used as a nonverbal mannerism to avoid or terminate stuttering.

- *Breathing patterns.* The stutterer may take in a deep breath or hold his breath in order to avoid or terminate stuttering.

The Cognitive/Emotional Aspects of Stuttering

Belief Systems. Now this section is a bit heavy on cognition, so bare with me as we wade through the swamp of beliefs. The cognitive aspects of therapy focus on the individual belief systems and how beliefs influence behavior change. Subsets of the concept of belief systems include the learning of irrational, erroneous beliefs (Meichenbaum, 1993), their impact on behavior and self-perception, modification of erroneous beliefs and self-perceptions through reality exposure, and the behavioral impact of self-dialogue based on a reconstructed self-reality. Bloodstein (1997) clarifies the point when he writes, "It is self-evident that if a stutterer could forget that he was a stutterer, this whole system of beliefs would vanish" (p. 170).

According to Rokeach (1972), there are five classes of beliefs in a belief system:

- Type A: Primitive Beliefs, 100% consensus.
- Type B: Primitive Beliefs, Zero consensus.
- Type C: Authority beliefs.
- Type D: Derived beliefs.
- Type E: Inconsequential beliefs.

Rokeach makes three basic assumptions: (1) Not all beliefs are equally important; (2) The more central the belief, the more it will resist change; (3) The more central the belief changed, the greater the impact on the rest of the belief system.

We first determine the client's critical beliefs, particularly the client's cognitive distortions about the stuttering. These beliefs form the basis of the client's interpretation, or erroneous beliefs, about the stuttering and it's impact on his life. For example, we are concerned with the stutterer's erroneous beliefs that when he stutterers people think he is retarded, that people laugh about the stuttering behind his back, that he is helpless to change the course of the stuttering, that therapy will not or is not having a positive effect, that there are many words that he cannot say under any conditions, and so forth. These beliefs, and others of this ilk, form the stutterer's paranoid, operative belief system. These are the beliefs that must be changed in the therapy process.

This belief system as a whole influences the cognitive set of the individual and is mainly based on the stutterer's interpretation of others' reactions to the stuttering. Although the stutterer may indeed misinterpret the listener's reaction to the stuttering, if the interpretation of the reaction is the foundation of a belief, it becomes a fact insofar as it is part of the stutterer's reality.

The negative belief system is reinforced through continual confirmation of the beliefs through the interpretation, or misinterpretation, of the behaviors of others. This forms the basis of the self-dialogue: a negative cognitive set that maintains the stuttering and the negative cognitive set itself.

Because the strongest beliefs are learned through negative experiences with the stuttering, any new positive belief to replace a negative one must be learned through positive experiences with the stuttering. This is the basis for building a new, positive belief system.

Grief Over Loss. The stutterer's belief system is directly related to his grieving over his loss (Kubler-Ross, 1969). What has the stutterer lost? He has lost the ability to speak like other people, to speak fluently. The five stages of grief are denial, anger, bargaining, depression, and acceptance. I have changed the last of these from "acceptance" to "resignation," because I do not feel that people who stutter ever "accept" the stuttering, but can, rather, "resign" themselves to the fact that they stutter.

When we apply these stages to the stutterer, we, and perhaps the stutterer, can gain some insight into why he thinks as he does. The stage of *denial* indicates that the stutterers are denying that their stuttering is a problem or that it will be with them the rest of their lives. To better understand how a stutterer can deny his problem, recognize that if one carefully analyzes the speech of any stutterer, he or she will find that a large majority of the speech is fluent. It is rare to find a stutterer who stuttered on more than 25% of the words spoken in all speaking situations. As mentioned earlier, even with the most severe stutterers, there are situations where speech is totally fluent. In light of this, it is not too difficult to imagine the stutterer denying he is actually a stutterer, or that it is a problem, or that it will be one for the rest of his life.

The second stage is *anger*, and most stutterers are angry. They are angry because they have lost the ability to speak fluently. They ask, "Why me?" They are looking for someone to blame for their affliction. They are angry with themselves for not having the courage to confront their stuttering and for allowing the stuttering to dominate their lives. They are angry because they cannot say what they want to say. There is also a lot of anger directed to listeners who, in their mind, respond negatively to them when they stutter by saying the word for them or looking away from them.

In the third stage, *bargaining*, the stutterer bargains in several ways. Some pray that the stuttering will be taken away in exchange for a commitment on their part to do something. As I related before, one client, a minister, prayed that if his stuttering was cured he would go into the ministry. He summarized the results of the bargain when he said that both he and God lost; he still stutters and God has a stuttering minister. The stutterer also bargains with the clinician. His bargain is that if he faithfully attends all the therapy sessions, the clinician will assume the responsibility for "curing" him of his stuttering.

The fourth stage is *depression*. The stutterer, after repeated attempts to free himself of the stuttering, finds that he cannot get rid of it and becomes depressed. This is a common emotion with all stutterers, especially those who have been through several therapy programs and still stutter.

The final stage is *acceptance/resignation*. Here, the stutterer finally resigns himself to the fact that he is and will always be a stutterer. He recognizes that there is no known cure for stuttering, but that appropriate therapy can help him by reducing the severity of the stuttering to the point where it is no longer a major negative influence in his life. He can then apply all the energy he wasted worrying about it to actively working on his speech in therapy.

Unfortunately, the stutterer does not progress through these stages and then settle into acceptance. He constantly goes back and forth through the stages but, as therapy progresses, he spends less and less time in the stages of denial, anger, bargaining, and depression. As the stutterer works his way through the various stages, there will be differing degrees of clinical resistance.

How Stuttering Begins

Stuttering has its roots essentially in childhood, most often beginning between 3 and 5 years of age (Bloodstein, 1975; Van Riper, 1982). It appears that the phenomenon may be related in some way to the normal dysfluencies that appear in the speech of younger children.

What begins as inconsequential repetitions and prolongations of sounds in the speech of a young child eventually becomes the main focus of attention in the speech of the child who is destined to stutter. As more attention is focused on the timing or phase errors in speech, the errors become the main focus of attention of the child. Once the child becomes aware of the errors in the flow of speech, he begins to focus more attention on the speech act, attempting to eliminate the errors. As the child becomes more sensitized to the interruptions in the flow of speech, he shifts his focus from ongoing speech, to phrases, to individual words, to syllables, to speech sounds and, finally, to basic movements associated with articulation, phonation, and respiration. The child is focused on the mechanics of speech, and the automaticity of his speech is now in jeopardy. The child is attending more to the mechanics of speech than to the content of the speech; because of this, the automaticity of speech is compromised, and the fluent flow of speech is interrupted by the first stages of stuttering.

In the most severe cases, the child is completely preoccupied with his struggle to complete each sound or movement. He is cognitively focused on every detail of his communication, be it tongue movements, phonation, breathing, mouth opening, and so forth. When and if the client reaches this point, he has lost most of the automaticity of the speech act.

The speech is now resplendent with secondary mannerisms; reactions which, when initially performed, prevented the stuttering from occurring. Although each performance of these behaviors temporarily eliminates the stuttering, they quickly lose their potency, and the stuttering, which had been eliminated by the behaviors, occurs once again. The client must then adopt another mannerism to prevent the stuttering from occurring. At some point in time, the stutterer makes the final adjustment between the mannerisms and the stuttering, settling on a procedure (verbal and/or non-verbal) that will provide, in his mind, a socially acceptable and somewhat dependable means of communication.

Where Stuttering Occurs

Now that we have some idea of what stuttering is, what behaviors are involved in the stuttering act, and how it develops, we should address the issues of where and when it occurs.

Physiologically. The repetition or prolongation can occur anywhere in the vocal tract where there is a point of articulation; that is, where two parts of the vocal tract come in contact during speech.

Phonetically. The block does not occur on the phoneme itself, but rather in the movement of the articulators from one position to the next. The block occurs in the transition between articulatory positions.

Linguistically. With normal speech, the speaker's attention is directed at merging thoughts into the ongoing act of speaking, where speech sounds, syntax, inflection patterns, and all other facets of oral communication are melded at a reflexive, automatic level. This normal cognitive activity is disrupted when the speaker's attention is diverted to listening for rhythm disruptions in the speech and subsequent attempts to prevent their occurrence through unique manipulations of the speech act.

It is at this crossroads where the stutterer must deal with his negative beliefs and his factual report of positive results. We are confronted with cognitive dissonance, where the client's expectation of failure (belief) is in direct conflict with his success. To resolve this conflict, the client's speech expectations must be raised to coincide with the improved speech performance. This is the clinical challenge; to change the negative cognitive set into a positive one based on new beliefs and the rejection of erroneous beliefs; to not allow the cognitive set to remain in a negative mode based on previously learned erroneous beliefs.

Socially. Stuttering occurs only in social environments. If the stutterer is alone, out of social contact, he will not stutter when he talks. However, when he is in a social environment, he is subjected to four general sources of communication stress, all of which increase the liklihood and severity of stuttering.

Degree of Propositionality. This source of communication stress involves how much thinking and talking the stutterer must do and how abstract the message is that he is attempting to communicate. A conversation such as a person asking the time of day has very little propositionality. But attempting to explain an abstract concept includes an inherently high degree of propositionality.

The Listener. This involves who the listener is, whether he is a figure of authority, a peer, or a person of the opposite sex, and how many listeners there are. All factors influence the amount of stress involved.

Emotional Content. What the stutterer talking about. This can be either a positive or negative emotion. If the person is explaining how he found a $100 bill, he will be excited and under the influence of positive emotion. But in trying to explain some noxious behavior of his, he would be influenced by negative emotion. Either type of intense emotional content will exacerbate stuttering.

Communication Stress. A good example of communication stress is speaking while under time pressure. This is commonly found while speaking on the phone. When you answer the phone, you are expected to talk immediately. When you are calling and a person answers, you are expected to respond as soon as the person answers. Almost all stutterers have some negative reaction to calling on and/or answering the telephone. With the telephone, there is no direct contact between the stutterer and his listener except through the speech, and this puts more intense demands on the speech production.

Techniques To Modify Stuttering Behaviors

Behaviors to Minimize Stuttering. It is important to note that our program is not fluency oriented, that is, we are not rewarding fluent speech. We reward the new speech behavior which, when performed, results in *controlled fluency.* The term *new speech behavior* is used to describe the way we will teach the client to speak. Actually, we will be changing four aspects of speech to achieve the new speech behavior. The four aspects we will be changing are referred to in the text as "REEF."

R—slower <u>rate</u> of speech;

E—attending to oral cues or <u>enunciation</u>;

E—<u>easy onset</u> of vocalization;

F—smooth <u>flow</u> of speech.

When the client performs his REEF, he is performing his new speech behavior, which results in controlled fluency. These aspects of speech are modified simultaneously, rather than one at a time. In other words, the new speech behavior is viewed as a behavior in and of itself. We will not deal with secondary mannerisms because they are only associated with stuttering blocks. If blocks do not occur, neither will the mannerisms. The four behaviors to change are as follows:

- *Rate of speech (R).* Our goal is a slightly slower rate of speech than normal, but not an exaggeratedly slow rate of speech. The speech rate should sound normal to the listener, although a bit slower than the speech rate of the average speaker.

- *Attending to oral cues (E).* The term "enunciation" is used to identify this step in therapy. This term is used because most clients understand what is meant by "enunciation." The enunciated speech should be slightly exaggerated with the mouth and lips being very active in speaking. If someone were to describe the fully enunciated speech, they might describe it as articulatate or precise.

- *Easy vocal onset (E).* The clients should be shown how to move the vocal folds from the open position to the phonatory position in a slow and deliberate fashion. In this way, the folds are prevented from closing beyond the phonatory position and moving into a locked, closed position. This technique is used in voice therapy to counteract the hard vocal attack.

- *Smooth flow of speech (F).* The flow of speech is extremely important in stuttering therapy. Almost all stuttering occurs when the individual begins speaking. If the speech is choppy, and the person must start speaking again each time he ends a short phrase or a word, he has a high probability of stuttering.

When asked how they know when the stutter occurred, the stutterer will report they hear it. In other words, they are "spectatoring" their speech, listening for the stuttering to occur. And this cognitive interference, listening for stuttering to occur, results in the breakdown of the automatic, reflexive nature of speech. This results in the fragmenting of the speech focus from concentration on context of the speech, down to attending to specific words, to syllables, to sounds, and eventually, to focusing on phonetic movements.

By refocusing the individual's attention on the enunciation, concentrating on the speech sounds, the spectatoring is minimized and the automatic and reflexive nature of speech is allowed to reestablish itself. Enunciation is, therefore, the keystone upon which fluency is based. Rate and flow are also important behaviors that encourage fluency, but function mainly as adjuncts to enunciation.

Behaviors to Terminate Blocks. We now turn to those behaviors that we introduce not to eliminate the stuttering, but to deal with stuttering blocks when and where they occur. These behaviors address one of the fears of the stutterer—how long the block will last once it occurs. There are two basic behavioral strategies the stutterer can turn to in order to terminate the block.

- *The glide*. The glide is the slow, purposeful, voluntary movement of the articulators from the initial position of the word (syllable) to the following vowel. This is a unique form of rate control, in that we are slowing down the specific movement of the articulators between the initial sound(s) and the following vowel. It is a slow and deliberate movement, which overrides the block. When introducing the glide, I first ask the client to tell me what the sounds are for the letters "b", "d", and "g." Almost without exception, the client will tell you "buh", "duh", and "guh." They introduce the neutral schwa vowel in order to produce the sound in isolation. The emphasis in the word should be on the correct vowel sound at the end of the glide.

- *Stop/correct*. This technique has a built-in danger of becoming a retrial, where the stutterer stops, backs up a few words, and tries to say the stuttered word again. We insist that the stutterer change his speech behavior when he uses this technique; that is, when he starts speaking again, he must emphasize his REEF. The block occurrs because he was not fully using his new speech behavior. When he starts again, using his REEF, the probability of the block occurring is greatly reduced. Great care must be taken to ensure that the stutterer does not just repeat the initial word or phrase, using the old speech behavior and performing a retrial.

Therapy Procedures for Adults and Children

The first thing we must address is the goal of stuttering therapy. We are really addressing two seperate goals, since the children who stutter are in a developmental stage of stuttering and the adults who stutter have progressed into confirmed stuttering or what Van Riper (1982) classified as secondary stuttering.

If we are working with a child who is in the beginning stage of stutterering, the clinical goal should probably be to cure the stuttering problem. And from my work with cognitive–behavioral therapy, it appears that most of the stuttering in children can achieve normal speech; that is, the stuttering can be permanently replaced by fluency.

With those children who cannot achieve fluency, even after numerous months of therapy, the therapist is faced with a choice: to continue with therapy, even though it is not achieving the desired end, or to dismiss the child from therapy. There is a third choice, though, and that is to shift the child's therapy into the adult phase, working with the child to control the stuttering, as the adult does in therapy. This would mean shifting the clinical goal from fluency to control.

As to the goal for the secondary stutterer, most members of our profession would agree that there is no cure for adult stutterers who have progressed to the secondary stage, or confirmed stuttering. So, if there is no cure, what is our goal? The semantic problem here is the word *fluent*. We seem to have divided stuttering treatment into the fluency paradigm and the control paradigm. And this introduces us to the concept of normal dysfluencies (as experienced by all human beings) and stuttering dysfluencies (those experienced only by people who stutter). Now, if this is interpreted correctly, people who stutter have both normal dysfluencies in their speech (because they are human beings) and stuttering dysfluencies (because they are stutterers). Thus, to hope to achieve total fluency (with no dysfluencies) is futile, since normal dysfluencies are part of normal speech. Because the stutterer is so preoccupied with fluency (they do not acknowledge or cognitively deal with normal dysfluencies), they can never achieve their dream, total fluency. So, the clinical goal with adult stutterers is to accept some stuttering, but reduce it to a minimum.

In presenting the therapy procedures for adults and children, several behavioral concepts appear in various sections of this book. When a special procedure or concept is used, for example the use of rewards and penalty, the usage is followed by the following symbolic reference. You can look up the reference in the index to find more information on the concept or procedure. In all therapy procedures, we are basing the interaction between the clinician and the client on the CIM. If you do not remember the concept, you can now look it up in the Index.

Therapy Procedures for an Adult Stutterer

Getting the New Behavior To Occur

The therapy interaction is directed at teaching the client the new behaviors of slower rate of speech, careful enunciation while speaking, using easy onset in speech, and the flow of words to eliminate unnecessary pauses. The behaviors can be taught using modeling, information, and guidance. As the new speech behavior occurs, rewards should be given to the client. With adult clients, rewards tend to be more verbal in nature and less materially oriented. It is the occurrence of the new behavior that is rewarded, not the resultant fluency. The fluency is only a by-product of the use of the new speech behavior.

The therapy interaction initially consists of the clinician demonstrating each behavior included in the REEF. As the client becomes more familiar with the new behaviors, the interaction changes from a teaching mode to a practice mode, where the clinician and client discuss various things while the client is using the REEF. The rewards provided for correct performance of the REEF are maintained as the client becomes more adept at melding the four new behaviors. He will also become more fluent, a by-product of the use of the new behaviors.

Stabilizing the New Behavior

The CIM continues to be the basis of clinical interaction. We are providing the client with an environment where he can practice the new speech behavior while speaking on a variety of topics. As we move into this phase of therapy, the performance of the new behavior is still dependent on the rewards the client receives in therapy. However, we now begin to slowly remove the rewards, changing our reward schedule from a continuous to an intermittent schedule.

The shaping process is still being used, although we are now shaping the new speech behavior to occur in different conversational modes and while speaking about different topics. We increase emotional content as the new behavior becomes more stable. We do not move out of this phase of therapy until the client can maintain his new speech, regardless of the topic in therapy, without prompts or rewards from the clinician. If the rewards are withdrawn too rapidly, the performance of the new behavior may slip. In this event, increase the rewards until the new behavior is stronger, and then begin to again remove the rewards, but withdraw them more gradually.

Generalizing the New Behavior

The new speech behavior is now occurring consistently, but not where needed, in talking situations outside of the therapy room. You must now transfer the new speech behavior to other talking environments. The focus of your therapy now shifts to the antecedent events, that is, the various $S+$ and $S-$ in the client's life. You will manipulate these stimuli so that new $S+$ encourages the new behavior to occur, and shift the $S-$ talking situations to either an $S0$ or an $S+$ to eliminate the negative effects of the $S-$. Therapy will focus on stimulus control.

You are still shaping the new speech behavior, but you are now concerned about its occurrence in situations with differing amounts of communication stress. Explain to the client that he will be able to use the new behavior in easier talking situations better than in more difficult ones. The most important aspect of therapy now is to develop some way the client can record his attempts to use the new speech behavior in outside talking situations.

You are now asking the client to give reports, written and/or oral, on how well he is able to use his new speech behavior outside the clinic room. Your stimulus to the client usually includes asking for information, but also giving needed information. For example, if the client has a problem with a high anxiety talking situation, you may provide him with information as to why he has difficulty with that situation. The interaction is highly cognitive, as the client discusses his talking experiences in other environments.

To record these attempts, you can use the logbook. You should make specific assignments as to the number of times you want him to practice his new behavior each day and instruct the client to start his practice in easier situations in order to increase the degree of success.

Maintaining the New Behavior

The time has come to gradually withdraw direct therapy contacts from the client. There should also be less and less input from us. You should allow the client to take more responsibility for his speech. He is not given answers to problems he might face, but is directed to plan a strategy to work through the problem, which you will discuss with him. The goal is to train him to be his own clinician, and we do this not by force or strategies, but by allowing him to think through the problem and to discuss it with us. We do not relate to him as a client, but more as a clinician discussing a client.

Therapy Procedures for Children Who Stutter

This therapy involves a lot of parental cooperation and a routine home program. To prepare the parent for the therapy, he or she should bring to the first therapy session a stack of poker chips, several small plastic bags for storage, and a container for the rewards the child will receive in therapy (aka "the store"). This program is based on a token economy where tokens (poker chips) are used as money to buy rewards from the store. During the initial session with the parent and the child, explain the store. Topics should include the following:

- What to buy as rewards: candy, cookies, small toys, etc.
- How to set the price for the rewards: one chip roughly equals one cent.
- When the "store" should be open: e.g., Tuesday and Friday evenings.

- The number of chips that can be earned per day at home: approximately 20 per day.
- The length of each session at home: approximately 10 minutes.
- Where the home session should be done: a quiet, private place in the home.
- The policy for saving chips: the client must buy something on each visit to the store, but he can also save chips for an expensive reward.

The rewards for the child are very important. These are the things that will motivate the child, and without motivation, therapy is all but useless. The higher the motivation, the quicker therapy will progress. Motivation is the *key* to successful therapy!

The goal of therapy with children is fluency, or normal speech. By the end of the third step in therapy you should achieve that goal. However, not all children will reach the level of normal speech. It is then up to you, the clinician, to decide whether to continue with therapy or stabilize the speech that the child has at this stage in therapy. Guidelines? I work with the children for approximately 3 months, seeing the child half an hour a week. The parent works with the child for about 10 minutes every day with the home program. At the end of 3 months, about 60% of the children achieve normal speech (i.e., fluency). The remaining 40% of the children achieve between 70% and 90% fluency. This therapy, like that for the adults, is based on the CIM.

Getting the Behavior To Occur

We start therapy with the child in a comfortable position and, through a story or conversation, get the child as relaxed as possible. You should model a general, relaxed manner, speaking slowly and using your lips to enunciate, i.e., "Easy Talking." Explain to the child how you are doing Easy Talking, using slow rate, enunciation, and flow. Use neutral topics as you talk to the child. You should also introduce your gestural cues in association with the slower rate of speech (a "slow down" hand gesture), the moving of the mouth for enunciation (a "move your lips" gesture), and the flowing of speech (a "flowing speech" gesture). The gestures you use will convey the message without interrupting the speech of the child.

When the child uses some of the Easy Talking behaviors and there is less stuttering, reward him verbally and with a token for the effort. Shape his speech toward more normal speech with the gradual elimination of dysfluencies through Easy Talking. When he is able to produce Easy Talking and achieve fluency consistently, move to the next phase of therapy. However, if the child uses secondary mannerisms when he talks (verbal or nonverbal) you may withhold the reward and explain to the child why he is not receiving the reward. Back off a bit at this point, lessening the stress on the child, and stay at that level until his fluency is reestablished before progressing again.

As you are working with the child, make certain the parent understands what you are doing in therapy. Model the goal behavior as you speak and ask the parent if there are any questions about what you are doing. You should give about 20 chips to the child in the therapy period (use one of the plastic bags), and this should be the quota in the home program as well. If you total these up, you will find that the child will earn about 160 chips a week, 140 from the parent and 20 from you. Lots of "money" to spend on rewards. Did I mention the fact that greed is a *powerful* motivating force!

The parents should open the store for the child twice a week. He can purchase anything he has the chips to buy, both from those you gave him or chips he earned from home. Remember, he can save chips for an expensive reward.

Stabilizing the New Behavior

You are now providing speaking environments so the child can practice Easy Talking on a variety of topics. The rewards continue for the use of Easy Talking and the resultant fluency. If the child begins to uses secondary mannerisms, return to the previous level of therapy and, moving slowly, shape the child's speech so he is back to current level without the secondary mannerisms.

Use a variety of topics for conversation. Keep track of the topics with which he has the most difficulty and, using your hand gestures for Easy Talking, try them again later in the same step in therapy. Keep rewarding the child for his successes in order to shape his speech toward fluency on all topics.

Generalizing the Behavior

The child should now be speaking quite fluently in therapy sessions with you and with his parent, but he will be somewhat dysfluent in his general speech out of the clinical environment. You are now going to consider the child's speech outside therapy, asking the child how he or she is talking in school, on the playground, with his friends, and so forth. You may want to establish a scale of success so the child can have a way of telling you how successful he is or how much stuttering occurs. Establish very good speech with you in therapy and then ask him to grade himself for that speech. In the therapy room with you in a relaxed situation, he should indicate that his speech is very good. Assign a level of fluency for this speech, using an A or a *1*. If you then increase the stress level of the conversation, he should begin to demonstrate more dysfluencies. This you would label a B or a 2 speech. Begin to ask him about other examples of his speech, e.g., when he is out on the playground with friends. He is likely not thinking about his speech at that time, so he should report less than a B or a 2. If you work at this, you can establish a means of communicating his level of speech in a variety of speaking situations.

In this final phase of therapy, you should phase out the reward system. He cannot depend forever on the rewards from the store for fluency. As you phase out the reward system from the store, you increase and strengthen the verbal rewards the child receives from you. Usually I set aside a treasured item in the store for the last reward, a reward for completing the therapy program.

In the event there is some regression later on with the child, the parent should reinstate the store and begin working again at the second stage of therapy, stabilizing the new behavior. The parent and the child are both familiar with the game, and it should go very rapidly to the generalizing of the new speech and termination of therapy. The following is some additional advice on working with young children:

1. Enjoy your young clients.

2. Use some humor with them.

3. Treat them as you yourself would like to be treated.

4. Have fun in therapy.

5. Laugh with them.

6. If you do these things in therapy, the children will enjoy you and your therapy! And if they enjoy their therapy with you, they will work hard at their goals. This is *motivation*!

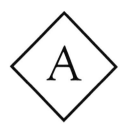

LEITH'S LAWS OF THERAPY

1. The probability that your therapy will be observed by a supervisor is directly related to your lack of preparation for therapy.

   Corollary:
   Your best therapy sessions are never observed by a supervisor.

   Corollary:
   The more disorganized your therapy session, the higher the probability you are being supervised.

2. Clients cancel or fail to appear for those therapy sessions you are best prepared for.

   Corollary:
   The probability of a client showing up for therapy is directly correlated with how poorly prepared you are for the therapy session.

   Corollary:
   The number of toys and games taken into a therapy session by a clinician is inversely related to her degree of preparation for therapy.

3. When a child becomes ill in therapy, the probability that he will throw up on you is directly related to how recently you had your clothes cleaned.

4. Children are the most hyperactive and difficult to control in therapy on those days you are not feeling well.

   Corollary:
   Children who you first judge will be pleasant to work with prove to be the most difficult clients you have.

Corollary:
Children are most difficult to control on the day their parents are observing therapy.

5. When your therapy is planned around a piece of equipment, it will be missing or not operating on the day you need it.

Corollary:
When you need a piece of clinical equipment for therapy, it will be checked out by the clinician just before you.

6. Your best ideas for therapy occur just after you have finished writing your therapy plan.

7. The last client of the day is always the one who needs the most clinical time.

8. The more difficult it is for you to get to work due to the weather, the more likely your clients will fail to appear for therapy.

Corollary:
Your client who misses the most appointments will keep his appointment on the day that you are absent because of illness.

9. Errors in client reports will not be noticed until the report is through its final typing.

10. When a clinical secretary is replaced, all files and final reports are lost for a period of no less than 2 months.

Postulate:
Clinical files disappear in direct relation to their importance.

11. Your late client will arrive for therapy immediately after you have poured yourself a cup of coffee.

Corollary:
When you go to get a cup of coffee during your only break in therapy for the day, the person just before you will have emptied the coffee pot.

12. You become a professional speech clinician only when the time you spend on paper work is equal to the time you spend in therapy.

13. When a piece of a test is misplaced, it remains lost forever.

Corollary:
Tests only lose their validity when more than 50% of the test is missing.

Corollary:
The first part of a test lost is the manual.

Corollary:
With tests consisting of forms and pieces to fit into the forms, the only thing left after 3 months are the pieces.

14. Lights are turned on behind one-way mirrors only when the client is looking into the mirror.

Corollary:
The time you decide to rearrange your clothes in the clinic room is that time when there are several observers behind the one-way mirror.

15. After all desirable rooms in an agency have been assigned, the speech clinician has the choice of all remaining space.

Corollary:
Speech clinical rooms must be located next to a bathroom, an elevator, a gymnasium, or a band rehearsal room.

16. Clinical equipment sent out for repairs never returns.

Corollary:
When equipment is returned from repairs, it still does not work.

17. Power cords used to connect clinical equipment to wall outlets disappear after 3 months.

Postulate:
Power cords that disappear are impossible to replace since no one manufactures a cord that matches the equipment.

18. If a piece of equipment operates on batteries, the batteries are always dead when you need to use the equipment.

19. When writing a diagnostic report from your notes, the data you most need will be on the piece of paper you threw away when you finished the evaluation.

20. The one cassette tape that jams in your recorder and is destroyed will contain your most important clinical recording.

Corollary:
The tape you use to record a general therapy session contained the language sample you worked 3 weeks to get.

Corollary:
When you finally get the language sample you wanted, you discover you forgot to push the "record" button on the tape recorder.

21. By the time you become aware of your young client's wiggling and squirming in his chair, it is most often too late.

> **Corollary:**
> The previous law applies 10-fold when you are holding the young client on your lap.

22. When school assignments are made for itinerant school speech clinicians, the older the clinician's car, the further apart the schools will be.

> **Corollary:**
> School assignments for itinerant clinicians are based on the longest possible drive from the clinician's home.

23. The day you wear a skirt to work will be the day your clients will require you to work on the floor with them.

> **Corollary:**
> On that day where you have worn a skirt and are working on the floor with your clients, you will have observers, most of whom are male.

24. When carrying your clinical materials to or from a clinic room, the item you drop will be the most fragile and the most expensive.

25. When you are late for a clinical appointment, your client will arrive twice as early as you are late.

26. When chocolate is used as a reward in therapy, clinicians give themselves more rewards than they give their clients.

27. Electrical outlets in clinic rooms are always located at the furthest point from the work table.

> **Corollary:**
> Power cords for tape recorders and audiometers are always six inches too short to reach the wall outlet plug.

> **Corollary:**
> All electrical extension cords disappear the day you need them.

28. The theories and therapies we were taught never apply to the clients with whom we are working.

> **Corollary:**
> Our specific clinical problems are never discussed in any journal or reference book.

29. Teenaged clients know more four-letter words than their clinicians.

> **Corollary:**
> Clinicians do not know most of the four-letter words the teenage clients use.

30. All adult chairs eventually end up in the children's therapy room.

    Corollary:
    The taller the clinician the higher the probability there will be only children's chairs in the therapy room.

31. When you ask another clinician to observe the problematic behavior of a client, he will behave perfectly during the observation.

32. When you are completely confident that your therapy is well planned and will go smoothly, the therapy will be a complete disaster.

33. When nothing else could go wrong with your therapy, it usually does.

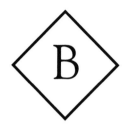

OPERATIONAL DEFINITIONS
OF CLINICAL BEHAVIORS

The following abbreviated descriptors are adapted from the *Handbook of Supervision: A Cognitive Behavioral System* (Leith, McNieve, & Fusilier, 1989). For complete descriptors, you are referred to the book.

Planning

1. Formulates Long-Term Goals

Long-term goals are those goals the clinician expects the client to achieve within a specific time frame (e.g., the goals expected to be reached during a semester in a clinical practicum). It is important to plan long-term goals when developing a treatment program for a client, because if the long-term goals are not established, the logical sequence of short-term goals cannot be formulated. It is important that the clinician, in formulating long-term goals, demonstrates insight and understanding of her client and the particular disorder being manifested. Goals should be comprehensive and appropriate for both the client and disorder.

2. Formulates Objectives Session by Session

The session objectives are a reflection of the clinical progress toward the long-term goals. The objectives should outline a logical sequence of clearly defined, measurable behaviors that are valid in relationship to the long-term goals. The clinician should state objectives in terms of client performance, using behavioral terminology and including methods to measure behavioral progress toward the objectives.

3. Modifies the Clinical Program When Change Is Indicated

The clinician's long-term and short-term planning typically centers around a particular clinical method or program. There are times when that method or program needs to be modified, and the clinician needs to be able to recognize when change is indicated. When the client's performance levels have reached a plateau and no further progress is being made with the present program, this should be a signal to the clinician to make the appropriate changes.

4. Materials Appropriate for Client

The choice of materials for therapy is an important consideration. The right materials can assist in creating interest in therapy and in achieving and maintaining approach motivation. However, if they are selected without considering the needs of the client and the type of disorder being worked with, the materials can work against the clinician by voiding any interest the client might have had and, perhaps, even by creating avoidance motivation.

5. Has Rationale for Clinical Procedures

There is no single clinical procedure for any type of client. Essentially, the clinician is free to use any clinical procedure she feels is appropriate for the client and the disorder. However, the clinician also needs to have a rationale for her selection of the procedure. The rationale should be based on factual information gathered from research findings, clinical reports, classroom lecture notes, conferences, or from some other reliable source. The clinician should also understand why the selected procedure will likely succeed with this particular client and disorder.

6. Structures Plan for Maximum Number of Responses

In order for learning to occur in the clinical environment, the client must be able to respond, to try to perform the behavior being taught, or to respond verbally to see if a new concept or skill has been learned. The more chances the client has to perform and practice the new behavior, the quicker learning occurs. The clinician's therapy plan should reflect this concept, making certain that the client has enough opportunities to respond.

7. Demonstration of Progress to the Client

In planning therapy, the clinician should always include some means of demonstrating progress to her client. In any learning situation, the learner must know where he is and where he needs to go to master the target behavior. He also needs to know of his progress as he moves closer and closer to achieving the goal. This awareness of progress is essential for interest and motivation, which are both essential for learning. This feedback keeps the learner on track, moving him step by step toward mastery of the goal behavior.

8. Significant Others Included in Therapy Plan

This may not apply with some adult clients where there is little reason to include significant others or where there are no significant others to include. However, in the main, with either adults or children, the clinician should plan to include significant others in some aspect of the therapy, be it for moral support during therapy or for carryover of the new behavior into external environments.

Interactions: Clinical and Supervisory

9. Sensitivity/Awareness

Throughout either the diagnostic or clinical session, the clinician needs to have a heightened awareness of the client. She needs to be sensitive to both direct comments by the client and to subtle clues that indicate interest, motivation, feelings, needs, and so forth. This information may be goal-related, indicating that the client is meeting an objective or that more instruction is needed. Or it may be related to how the client is feeling, physically or emotionally.

10. Relates to the Client as a Person

In a humanistic approach to therapy, the clinician treats her client as a human being and not, as in a technical or mechanical approach, as a subject in an experiment. The clinician should relate to her clients with dignity and respect, demonstrating unconditional positive regard. If the clinician interacts with an adult aphasic client as she would with a child, this will have an adverse effect on the client's attitude toward therapy. The clinician should also demonstrate to the client that she is sincerely interested in the client as an individual, not just interested in the communication disorder. Her focal point in the clinical interaction is on the client, not on the clinical procedure, method, or strategy.

11. Positive Affect in Therapy

The clinician should recognize that her attitude or cognitive set in a clinical interaction will have a direct influence on the attitude or cognitive set of the client or significant other. If she is enthusiastic about what she is doing, others coming in contact with her will more than likely also be enthused. She should appear to enjoy the experience, and chances are her client will too. She should demonstrate sincerity in her relations with her client or his significant others by exhibiting a relaxed and caring attitude in the clinical setting.

12. Negative Personal Factors Removed from Therapy

The secret to good interpersonal relations is to keep one's own negative feelings and personal problems from interfering with the relationship. We can only do this by making a concerted effort to block them from surfacing. The clinician should keep her personal attitudes, feelings, and beliefs out of her clinical interactions. The most important thing is that she recognize her own biases. If she does not recognize and then control her personal biases, they will show in her interactions with her clients. If her biases are negative, her relationships will deteriorate to the point where therapy is impossible.

13. Initiative/Independence

The end result of supervision should be self-supervision. The foundation of self-supervision is initiative and independent problem solving by the clinician. When problems or questions arise, the clinician should demonstrate self-initiative and make an attempt to find answers before seeking help from the supervisor. She should have alternative solutions prepared when going in for a supervisory conference. As the clinician gains knowledge and experience, she should become more independent in both recognizing problems and seeking solutions.

14. Confident Image in Clinical Setting

When a person is involved in working with others in any helping profession, the recipient of the aid must have confidence in the individual providing the aid.

Confidence and credibility go hand in hand, and clinical credibility is an essential part of therapy. Hence, the clinician should make a positive professional impression on her clients and their significant others. She should instill confidence in them, confidence that she is a competent clinician and knowledgeable about the diagnosis and treatment of the client's particular communication disorder.

15. Response to Supervision

Supervision must, by definition, concentrate on both the positive and the negative aspects of whatever is being supervised. There are no problems with the praise a clinician receives for good performance; only the negative comments have the potential to create problems. Yet, it is the modification of the weak or incorrect behaviors that improves the overall performance of the supervised activity and the skills of the clinician. The clinician should view her supervisor as her clinical teacher, not as an adversary, and she must accept constructive criticism without becoming defensive.

16. Informing Client/Significant Others

When parents or significant others are involved, either directly or indirectly, in the treatment program of a client, it is their right to know what is transpiring. The clinician should keep parents and significant others informed about the client's progress in therapy. The information should be presented in an organized manner and without the use of professional jargon.

17. Interactions With Other Professionals

In almost any clinical program, the clinician will find herself interacting with other professionals. She should interact with these individuals in a professional manner, and she should reflect self-confidence. She should speak, dress, and behave in a professional manner.

Management

18. Record Keeping

In any professional setting, it is critical that complete records be maintained on clients. This may be for insurance purposes, attendance records, legal protection, billing procedures, tracking clinical progress, or any number of other reasons. It is the responsibility of the clinician to start and maintain these records. Perhaps the most essential records are those kept on a session-to-session basis for each individual client. Without these records, clinicians are hard pressed to remember specific details about each client, such as which techniques are being used and how well the client is doing in terms of learning a new behavior. Effective therapy is dependent on such records.

19. Stimulus Control

In the operant model, responses originally occur without a stimulus, and their future performance is dependent on the consequence of their occurrence—a reward or a penalty. However, when another stimulus, such as the person administering the contingent event, becomes associated with the reward or penalty, it becomes a discriminative stimulus, either a positive discriminative stimulus ($S+$) or a negative discriminative stimulus ($S-$). These stimuli can be manipulated in a number of ways in order to enhance therapy. Negative stimuli can be reduced, positive stimuli can be increased, the roles the stimuli play can be changed so that an $S-$ becomes an $S+$, and so forth. This control over and manipulation of the stimuli is essential for effective and efficient therapy.

20. Management of Client Behavior

If a client exhibits disruptive or manipulative behaviors in the therapy/evaluation session, clinical progress is seriously hampered. The inappropriate behaviors may be as extreme as running around the therapy room, yelling, or throwing things, to more subtle manipulation such as constantly talking about other things to keep the focus off the difficult tasks in therapy. The question that arises here is who is in control of the therapy/diagnostic session. The clinician should establish this control factor very early in therapy, probably during the first clinical meeting with the client. If the clinician fails to address disturbing and distracting behaviors, clinical progress will be minimal, since therapy time is wasted in attempting to get control of the client and have him attend to the clinical tasks.

21. Client Motivation and Attention

Motivation is the state of need or desire within an individual that activates that person to try to satisfy that need or desire. The clinician cannot directly motivate her client or significant other, but she can manipulate important fac-

tors influencing motivation so that it is more apt to occur. These factors include such variables as interest, concern, success, and relevant reward or
penalty. With these in mind, the clinician can direct her therapy or conference
so that the probability for motivation to occur is greatly enhanced. Without
motivation, clinical progress will be at a minimum.

Procedures

22. Clinical Goals Clear to the Client

Any developmental process is enhanced if the person involved in the process
knows its purpose and what it will produce. Just as we believe a clinician
should set goals with the supervisor and understand the expectations, we feel
the effectiveness and efficiency of therapy can be increased if the client
knows what is expected of him and where therapy is going. Therefore, the
clinician should make the clinical goals, both long-term and short-term,
known to the client. Each session should be started with a clear statement of
the goals for the particular session. The clinician should also make sure the
client knows what behaviors he needs to perform in order to meet those
goals. Periodically throughout the session and at the end of the session, the
clinician should verify that the client understands the clinical task and the
goals.

23. Goal-Oriented Therapy

The session goals should remain in focus throughout the clinical interaction,
with all activities designed to elicit goal-related behavior. The clinician should
guard against getting off-track. At times, the client may want to talk about
other things, and it may be important for him to do so. But as soon as possible,
attention should be directed back to the task at hand. The clinician, too, may
be tempted to stray from the target learning as opportunities for learning other
factors arise. She should resist the temptation and remain on target.

24. Use of Materials and Activities

No matter how well designed or well intended teaching materials and activities are, their effectiveness is directly related to how they are used in the
learning environment. The best clinical materials can be rendered useless
by inept and inappropriate use. If an activity designed for one purpose is
used for a purpose for which it was never intended, its effectiveness is

diminished. The clinician should not only be careful in her selection of materials and activities for her therapy, she should also be accomplished in their use.

25. *Effectiveness of Instructional Techniques*

There are many techniques and strategies that can be used to teach. However, their effectiveness and efficiency depend on the particular type of teaching being done and on the individual being taught. Techniques and strategies must be selected carefully to meet effectiveness and efficiency criteria. Regardless of reports on the effectiveness and efficiency of a technique or strategy, if it is not used properly, it is worthless. The clinician should, in selecting techniques and strategies for her therapy, carefully select those that are applicable to her particular teaching task and the individual client's learning style.

26. *Evaluating Responses*

In any learning situation where an individual is attempting to substitute one behavior for another, the change cannot be accomplished unless the individual recognizes when each behavior occurs and can differentiate between them. Therefore, if a client is to substitute a new speech behavior for the old, incorrect speech behavior, he must be able to recognize when each behavior occurs. And if he is to learn this, he is taught this skill by the clinician. The first requirement is that the clinician must be able to discriminate between the two behaviors correctly and consistently. If she is confused between the performances, she will not be able to teach the client to differentiate. And if the client cannot differentiate, there will be no extension of the new behavior outside the therapy environment.

27. *Time Efficient Procedure*

There are many teaching procedures, but some are more efficient than others. We might consider two procedures that are equally effective in that they accomplish the same goal. However, one procedure takes one week and the other takes one month. Since the two procedures are equal in effectiveness, we make our choice based on the efficiency of the process. If therapy is to be time efficient, the clinician must select efficient procedures. The clinical process must be time efficient so the behavior change goal may be reached within the shortest period of time.

28. Clinical Flexibility

If we are using a particular strategy to solve a problem and we find that the strategy is not appropriate or we are not making any headway with the problem, we change to another strategy we think is better fitted to solving the problem. If the client is not making any progress in therapy, we should evaluate the procedures we are using and make changes if necessary. However, in order to do this the clinician must be perceptually involved in the therapy process. She must be aware of the changing attitudes, feelings, or needs of her client.

29. Use of Modeling, Information, Guidance, and Feedback

The teacher's main tool in teaching any activity is the stimulus that she presents to the learner. This is that part of the learning process where the clinician presents the new behavior along with a variety of instructions on how the learner can perform it. The clinician's stimulus in therapy is made up of modeling, information, and guidance in various combinations. She primarily uses the auditory and visual sensory channels to present her stimulus, but also is free to use the bodily sense channel with various forms of guidance. By manipulating the stimulus through assorted combinations of modeling, information, guidance, and the sensory channels involved, the clinician can adjust the stimulus, making it more appropriate for the individual client. If the clinical stimulus is not appropriate for the client, therapy is not effective since the client does not understand what is expected of him. Once the client has attempted to perform the behavior, he must have specific feedback about the correctness or incorrectness of the attempt. This reflects the opinion of the clinician. It may be interpreted as a reward or penalty, but it should be more closely allied with providing information about a completed behavioral performance.

30. Use of Reward and Penalty

The selection of pleasant and aversive contingent events, rewards, and penalties in an operant paradigm is a very challenging task. At best, these are selected on the "best guess" of the person making the selection. These events can only be verified as rewards and penalties according to their effects on the frequency of occurrence of the behaviors to which they are applied. The reward and penalty selected by the clinician must be appropriate to the individual client. The reward and penalty must also be appropriate for the clinical setting (e.g., university clinic, hospital clinic, private agency). The reward and penalty contingency must be carefully maintained, and the reward schedule of presentation must be appropriate for the stage of therapy it is being applied in (i.e., continuous reward for fast learning early in therapy). Because the strength and effectiveness of rewards and penalties can change rapidly, the clinician must continue to monitor their effects and, if they are no longer functioning as they should, change to another pleasant or aversive contingent event. The clinician should also be aware of satiating a client with a reward so as to avoid having to change rewards during therapy.

31. Client Self-Evaluation

After learning how to perform a new behavior, such as a new way of holding a tennis racket, the individual must begin to use the behavior in its normal environment. In order to do this, the individual must learn to monitor and evaluate the behavior as it is occurring. This self-evaluation then makes it possible for the individual to use the new behavior in its normal environment or to modify the old behavior when it occurs. This self-evaluation is an important behavior that must be taught in the clinical program. For new behaviors to occur outside the clinical environment, the client needs to learn how to evaluate his behavioral performance. Only after there is self-evaluation can self-correction occur. The clinician should encourage this by modeling the desired behavior and encouraging the client to imitate the model. When self-evaluation does occur, the clinician should reward the behavior in order to increase the probability that the self-evaluation behavior will occur again. The clinician's therapy plan should reflect self-evaluation as a clinical goal, and there should be methods and strategies included to teach this behavior.

32. Client Talking/Response Time

In a learning situation where behavioral rehearsal is an important part of the learning process, time must be allowed for the behavioral rehearsal to occur. The rate of learning will be directly related to the amount of time allocated for rehearsal. In order to learn a new speech behavior, the client must practice it in the clinical environment. The clinician should structure her therapy so the clinical activities elicit a maximum number of behavioral responses from the client. The clinician's talking time should be aimed at providing modeling, feedback, and attempts to elicit more responses from the client. Talking time is structured for the client, not the clinician. The client needs time to respond to the clinician in the clinical environment.

33. Behavioral Data Collection

In order to determine if learning is taking place and to evaluate the efficiency of the teaching methods, an instructor must establish a behavioral performance baseline and then follow this up with either periodic or continuous data collection to compare with the baseline data. This is the most efficient way to chart learning progress. The clinician needs to develop a recording system so she has a continuous record of both the correctness and the frequency of occurrence of the target behavior. This is part of the clinician's cognitions in every clinical transaction. Without this data there is no way of charting progress. If the correctness of the response is not increasing, she should adjust her clinical stimulus. She should also check her reward and the schedule of presentation she is using. Knowing the percentages of correct responses allows her to know when the objective is too difficult or when it has been met so as to move on to another objective.

34. Session Goals Remain in Focus

In some clinical sessions, there may be more than one objective. In this instance, the clinician must not ignore one goal when she focuses therapy on the second goal. In other words, regardless of the number of clinical objectives there are in a session, the clinician must maintain some clinical attention on all clinical objectives.

Diagnosis

35. Test Administration

All tests have a standard administration procedure, and if the test is to be valid, it must be administered according to its protocol. The examiner should give all instructions clearly and concisely, making sure the client understands the instructions. All basals, ceilings, and thresholds should be established correctly, and the tests should be scored or marked according to the test protocol. Tests are only as valid and reliable as the administrative procedure used to administer them.

36. Clinical Observation Skills

Observational skills are basic to assessments of performance. Much information is gleaned from observations of the individual being assessed, and this information supplements the information from more formal assessment procedures. The clinician should be sensitive to and aware of all relevant client behaviors or behaviors of significant others. This would include not only what is said or done but also how it was said or done. The clinician should observe carefully all of the client's behaviors in the diagnostic situation, including both those behaviors being assessed in the diagnostic session and the client's general behaviors in that situation. In many instances, these general behavioral observations will provide a valuable supplement to the behavioral data collected in the formal tests, yielding a more accurate and complete diagnosis.

37. Test Interpretation and Recommendations

Tests of any kind are only as valuable as the way they are interpreted. If the test results are not interpreted correctly or thoroughly, the value of the diagnostic examination is lost. The clinician should take great care in interpreting the results of any tests that have been administered since recommendations will be based on these findings. Interpretation of formal tests should include the clinician's observations of client behaviors. She needs to consider her clinical observations as she evaluates test results and makes recommendations.

38. Professional Report Writing

Things are written so that there is a permanent record, a record that can be reviewed repeatedly over time. Professional reports may be read by a variety of persons involved with a client, including other professionals as well as significant others. The report should be written in such a way as to convey information about the client to the reader. The information is provided so others involved with the client can plan their own intervention program or work with you in resolving the client's problem. The report should be well organized, written without jargon, and grammatically correct. All information contained in the report should be pertinent to the client's problem, accurately reported, and stated clearly and concisely.

Additional Clinical Responsibilities

39. Observes Clinical Rules

Rules are made to preserve order. Without rules, chaos would reign. Clinic or agency rules are necessary to maintain an orderly, professional operation in any clinical program. Because there are so many people involved in a clinical operation, it is extremely important that rules are understood by all persons involved so there is a constant flow of information, continual updating of client data, properly maintained appointment schedules, and so forth. The clinician should be familiar with all clinical rules, policies, and procedures and should follow these guidelines in all her professional dealings within the clinic. This has a lot to do with professional responsibility.

40. Prepares for Clinical Conferences

Teachers like to have their student read the assignments prior to the classroom contact so that the student is prepared for and can participate in the class. In the same vein, when a clinical conference is arranged, the clinician should prepare for the conference by reviewing all pertinent information about her therapy and bringing the information with her to the meeting. Her review of the information should result in clinical questions for the supervisor as well as independent thoughts about how to improve her therapy. It is advisable for the clinician to write these questions prior to the conference. If she is an advanced clinician, she should be prepared for an indirect supervisory approach where she will enter into discussions about her therapy with her supervisor.

41. Contributes Alternative Procedures

In preparing for the supervisory conference, the clinician should develop alternative clinical plans for semester or session goals and the procedures to be used to meet those goals. She should also bring in recommendations designed to adequately meet the client's needs and enhance the treatment procedures. In all cases, the alternative clinical plans should be behaviorally oriented and based on the client's performance in both the clinical and outside environments.

42. Written Work Is Professional

All written work, including diagnostic reports, sessions plans, special reports, and other assigned papers, should be carefully written. Sentence structure, spelling, and grammar should be given particular attention. Professional terminology should be used when appropriate, but not to the point where the report or paper is difficult for a layperson to understand. The key word for written work is clarity. All written work should follow the established guidelines and time specifications of the clinic.

43. Self-Supervision of Clinical Performance

Although this is the last of the clinical behaviors deemed essential for satisfactory clinical performance, it is perhaps the most important one. Self-supervision is essential if there is to be professional growth beyond the supervised clinical experience. The entire supervision program is focused on training the clinician to be able to supervise herself and demonstrate clinical problem solving. She should readily recognize and identify those behaviors that facilitate and/or interfere with clinical success. She should also plan a program for improving her clinical skills that includes both setting forth behavioral goals and implementing a program where these goals can be achieved.

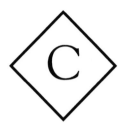

LEITH'S WMEOANRINDGSS

1. TEETH   TEETH

2. PIT
   CH

3. MUCOUS
   CLEFT

4. **TONGUE**

5. NASAL L
        E
        A
        K

6. (LIP, LIP) "AH"

7. NODE
   CORDS

8. MANNERISMS, *mannerisms*

9. PECTORALIS
   pectoralis

10. I
    N
    F
    L
    E
    C
    T
    I
    O
    N

11. V O W E L
      O   E
      W   W
        E O
      L V

12. TENVOCALSITY

13.   L
     N   O
    O   C
     I U
       T

R
E
I
N
14. REINFORCER
O
R
C
E
R

15. MISSED • MENT

16. RESONANCE
GLOTTAL

17. SEYRNRTOARX

18. WORD + FINDING =

19. NORMAL WITH LIMITS

20. R   I   L   I
A   C   T   N
T   U   A   O

21.   M
E   T
S
P
U

22.   U
V
U
L
A

NOTE: The answers to the word games in Chapter 3 are as follows:
1. Cleft palate
2. Up in pitch
3. Multiple artic errors
The answers to the WMEOANRINDGSS above are given below. They are upside down so you cannot cheat and look ahead. You will also find out the hidden meaning of WMEOANRINDGSS in this section.

Answers to WMEOANRINDGSS: (1) space between teeth, (2) pitch break, (3) submucous cleft, (4) macroglossia, (5) post-nasal drip, (6) bi-labial sound, (7) node on the cords, (8) secondary mannerisms, (9) pectoralis major and minor, (10) falling inflection, (11) vowel triangle, (12) vocal intensity, (13) circumlocution, (14) positive reinforcer, (15) missed appointment, (16) supra glottal resonance, (17) error in syntax, (18) word finding problem, (19) within normal limits, (20) distorted articulation, (21) deviated septum, (22) bifid uvula. You must look for the hidden meaning in words.

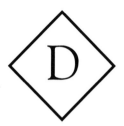

PLANNING AND DISCUSSING PROBLEM SOLVING

There are no standard answers to the following situations. What follows are my interpretations of the clinical problems and how I might approach them. You may indeed have a better approach. This section is meant as an exchange of ideas, so compare my answers with yours and try to determine why there are differences.

Chapter 7

Situation A

The 17-year-old boy presents several problems as we attempt to determine what an appropriate stimulus will be. Our first consideration must be the influence of the possible hearing loss on his perception of the sound in the words we are trying to teach him. Our clinical goal is to teach him a basic vocabulary that others in his environment can understand. If his hearing loss is so severe that our model of a word is extremely distorted, he may produce the word in such a fashion that it still cannot be understood by others; this should be the first test. We may also find that the hearing loss is not a significant influence. We might get some distortion, but the listener can still identify the word.

If there is too much distortion in the auditory channel, we might supplement auditory input with physical guidance of the oral structures in the production of the word. We may even have to break the words down into individual sounds and teach them through a combination of modeling and physical guidance.

We do not have any information about the cognitive function of this client, but we are suspicious because there is a history of brain injury. Both the modeling and physical guidance call for cognitions on the part of the client. If the modeling and physical guidance fail to produce the correct response, we might then add some verbal guidance, giving the client some hints about how he might change his speech attempt to make it correct. As a last resort, we might add behavioral information, but this requires a rather high cognitive level.

With this client, we want to avoid as much as possible our dependence on the auditory channel and high cognitive function. These are the two factors that are most suspect. Therefore, we turn to stimuli that are more visually or physically oriented.

Situation B

The 45-year-old laryngectomized client poses some very interesting problems. First of all, how are we going to teach esophageal speech? We can provide behavioral information to the client, but this is all very abstract. How can we verbalize production of this form of speech? It would be better if we provided a model at first so the client can see and hear what we are doing in order to produce the "voice." After the client has seen and heard the model, the behavioral information is much more meaningful. This is why it is so very important that the speech clinician be able to perform all the special behaviors she is asking her client to perform. Without the model, the learning process is going to be very slow and frustrating. We are already dealing with a client who is depressed, and he does not need any additional frustration. We can supplement the model and the behavioral information with verbal and physical guidance as the client attempts to produce esophageal speech. Still, the most important stimulus is the model of esophageal speech.

The client is depressed and this has a negative influence on therapy. We can use both general and behavioral information to attempt to offset the depression. We provide the client with information about others who have had a similar operation who have then gone on with a successful career. We give the client positive statistics and facts about the disorder. We can also approach the depression by using our contingent events. There is nothing better to ward off depression than success. And success is even sweeter when there is a meaningful reward associated with it. We must plan the therapy carefully so that the client is successful. He must see that he is able to succeed in modifying the disability, and then he must receive a meaningful reward.

Situation C

What do we do with a 7-year-old who has everything? We will find it very difficult to work with approach motivation to achieve something. We are probably going to have to turn to avoidance motivation with this child. We are going to have to find something she wants to avoid and then cultivate her avoidance motivation. Our contingencies are going to be penalty oriented and her reward will be to avoid the penalty, a negative reward. For example, let us say that the child enjoys playing a certain game with us in therapy. We tell the child that we will play this game at the end of each therapy session, but she will have to "buy" the game so we can play. We then give her 10 tokens and say, "Here is some special kind of money we will use to 'buy' the game. You have 10 tokens, and the game costs 7 tokens. You can 'buy' the game with the tokens you have. But we have to learn a new sound first, and if you are not paying attention to me, I will take a token away from you. If you do not have 7 tokens at the end of our speech work, you cannot 'buy' the game, and we will not be able to play." This is "response cost," where her nonattending responses cost her a token.

There is also the chance that we could use the game for approach motivation if she really wants to play it. In this event, we would reward her for attending to therapy. She would be told that she would have to have a certain number of tokens in order to "buy" the game so we could play. We would then give her tokens for attending to therapy. This token economy is reward-oriented, while the previous one is penalty-oriented.

There is also the possibility that we can combine rewards and penalties. In this token economy we would reward attending behavior and penalize the nonattending behavior. This might be the best approach we could use, since it would both encourage attending behaviors (approach motivation) and discourage nonattending behaviors (avoidance motivation).

Situation D

In order to teach this 9-year-old boy to produce easy vocal onset (easy vocal attack), we should provide him with a model. This means that clinicians must be able to perform this behavior. We select a single vowel sound and produce it with a hard and an easy vocal onset so the client can hear the difference in production. We then ask him to attempt to imitate the easy vocal onset. If his attempt is close to the model, we may be able to shape it by providing him with some guidance, primarily verbal and gestural. We might tell him to make the transition into the vowel slower and indicate this by a hand gesture. We could also repeat the model, slowing down the behavior so he can hear how we gradually introduce vocalization.

What would we do if we could not produce the behavior ourselves? We would have to depend on behavioral information. We would explain carefully how to produce easy vocal onset. This could be accomplished by telling him to start with an [h] sound and then move into the vowel. If we had selected the [ei] vowel, we would tell him to say the word "hay" very slowly. The next step would be to gradually reduce the duration of the [h] sound until, for all practical purposes, it no longer exists and the [ei] vowel is produced with easy vocal onset. During the course of shaping the easy vocal onset, we would also use guidance, both verbal and gestural. The only thing missing here is our model of easy vocal onset. However, we could use this same technique to train ourselves to produce the easy vocal onset behavior. There really is no reason why we cannot provide a model of this behavior. Speech clinician, heal thyself.

Before we close this case, let us consider what other things we would do to reduce the amount of vocal abuse that is occurring. If we decided that we also wanted to alter the habitual pitch, we would again use modeling, guidance, and information as we changed the pitch of the voice. In terms of other forms of abuse, such as too much yelling and shouting, we would rely primarily on information about how this injures the vocal folds. In other words, we would give the client a lecture on vocal hygiene and hope that this would have an impact on his use of the voice. We attempt to influence this client's attitudes and beliefs regarding the use of his voice. This is basically a form of counseling, and it takes the form of changing the client's cognitive set about how he views his voice. There is an exchange of attitudes and beliefs between us. We must first of all determine how he views his voice before we can attempt to change his views. This is only one of many clinical situations in which we have to work on the client's cognitive set as well as on speech behaviors.

Chapter 8

Situation A

The removal of the prompt from this 50-year-old client should not pose any serious problems if we do it gradually. If we suddenly remove the prompt, the word may indeed fail to occur, so we remove it in gradual stages. Let us suppose that the gestural guidance prompt is to pretend to drink water from a glass. The prompt consists of our pretending to pick up a glass, lift it to our mouth, and then tilt it up so we can drink from it. We can gradually remove the prompt by eliminating the final step, the tilting of the glass. We can even gradually remove the last step by not tilting the glass as far, or not moving our head back as far. We remove the prompt in steps small enough that the client can maintain the response as the prompt is removed. We shorten the duration of the stimulus by making each successive prompt less complete. With some clients, we may be able to remove the prompt in large steps, while with other clients we have to create very small steps.

Situation B

Our problem with the 13-year-old client with cerebral palsy is that we moved too fast when we went from a continuous reward to a 2:1 ratio. We suddenly reduced the presentation of the reward to 50% of occurrences of behavior. It would be much better if we changed the ratio of reward more slowly. Our first step might be to go to a 10:9 ratio, rewarding 9 occurrences and then passing over the 10th performance. When the behavior is maintained with this ratio we can reduce it to 10:8, then 10:7, and so forth. After we have reached the 1:1 ratio, we can shift to a 2:1 ratio, where he is rewarded for every other production. This can continue through 3:1, 4:1 ratios, and so forth, until the reward is eliminated and the behavior continues to occur.

Situation C

The 15-year-old boy who is going through voice change is reacting to peer pressure, and we must help him through this difficulty. We should deal with it while he is still in the clinical environment so we can control the variables in the speaking situations. Role playing can be used with this client. We can start by having him use his new pitch while pretending to talk to a person who is not threatening to him. We can play the role of the other person. We can then work our way up through more intimidating people. This might be followed by having another client come into the clinical room to talk with the client. Then we might bring in a couple of other clients. We gradually introduce those talking situations where the client is afraid to, or cannot, produce the new pitch. As the client is successful with the talking situations in the clinical environment, he will experience less tension and more confidence in those talking situations in the external environment. The gradual presentation of these talking situations helps the client generalize the behavior to environments outside the clinic room.

Chapter 9

Situation A

We face a couple of problems in attempting to generalize the new speech of our 67-year-old laryngectomy client. He is depressed about the effects his speech will have in his social contacts and, since he is a widower, he has no support system to help him generalize his speech to other environments. First of all, we should have dealt with the social impact of his speech earlier in therapy. We will have to deal with this· by giving him general information about others with his condition. We might even arrange to have someone who has had a laryngectomy visit the client and talk about how he has adjusted. The introduction to another person with the same condition does wonders for morale.

The other problem we face is the lack of a support system. With no wife in the picture, we could ask about his close friends. He may have some friends with whom he meets on a regular basis. Perhaps they meet daily to play cards or some other activity. We might ask our client if he would bring a close friend with him to therapy. We could then formally, or informally, create an S+ for our client by shifting the stimulus role of the friend. The formal creation of an S+ could only be done if the client agrees to it. We would explain that his friend could help him remember to use the new speech, and he could also tell the client how well he was speaking. Again, we must remember that our client can use esophageal speech but only in the clinic room. If we can introduce some of our client's friends into the treatment program, we can create a support system and get the new speech to occur in other environments.

Situation B

Our 14-year-old girl is not only dealing with a voice disorder; she is dealing with puberty and peer pressure. Fortunately, she has a support system because her parents are concerned and willing to help. She is caught in something of a "trap" situation. If she uses her old voice, people laugh or tease her about it. At the same time, if she uses her new voice, she is often teased because the voice is so different. All this is going on during those sensitive, early teenage years. One would think that the new voice would be so pleasing that she would use it immediately in other environments, but there are ambivalent emotional factors that pull her in two directions.

Since we have the cooperation of her parents, we should start introducing the new voice in a highly controlled environment, the home. We will shift the roles of the parents to that of an S+ by having them give her verbal praise when the new voice occurs. We should be able to establish the new voice in this environment without too much trouble because we have the cooperation of the parents. Our next step would be to have our client bring a friend home and use the new voice with her friend in this structured environment. We could then increase the number of friends brought into the home, controlling the gender makeup of the group. If our client feels more comfortable with female friends, we might start increasing the number of girls in the group. Boys could be introduced either as members of the group of friends or as a single male friend brought to the house. As we gradually introduce the new voice into our client's environment, she will not experience the tension that prevents her from producing the voice in outside situations.

Situation C

Our approach to this 65-year-old man with a receptive language problem would be quite similar to the one we used with our 14-year-old voice client. We must gradually introduce other talking situations in order to allow the client to gain confidence. We are fortunate in this instance, because the new behavior is occurring in the home environment. We strengthen this circumstance by making our client's wife a very strong $S+$ through a heavy reward program.

We then gradually modify the home environment by bringing in other people. We might start with a close friend and carefully control the content of the conversation to prevent it from getting too abstract. The topics of conversation would then be varied in order to increase the demands on comprehension. The number of friends brought into the house would then be gradually increased and the topics of conversation controlled as before.

As our client is gaining confidence in the home, we would instruct our client's wife to take him along on her various shopping trips and while doing errands. We would instruct our client to enter into small conversations with people in these different environments. Because his wife is with him and is a strong $S+$, she will cue appropriate behaviors to occur and will provide much needed moral support for our client. She will also be able to intervene if a conversation begins to become threatening to our client. We are again introducing threatening situations in a controlled fashion, making certain that our client can succeed and gain confidence in these situations.

REFERENCES AND
RECOMMENDED READINGS

Anderson, J. L. (1988). *The supervisory process in speech–language pathology and audiology.* San Diego: College-Hill.

Bandura, A. (1969). *Principles of behavior modification.* New York: Holt, Rinehart & Winston.

Barlow, D. H. (1988). *Anxiety and its disorders: The nature and treatment of anxiety and panic.* New York: Guilford.

Beck, A. T. (1976). *Cognitive therapy and the emotional disorders.* New York: International University Press.

Bloodstein, O. (1975). *A handbook on stuttering.* Chicago: National Society for Crippled Children and Adults.

Bloodstein, O. (1997). Stuttering as an anticipatory struggle reaction. In R. Curlee & G. M. Siegel (Eds.), *Nature and treatment of stuttering: New directions.* Needham Heights, MA: Allyn & Bacon.

Bloomer, H. (1956). Professional training in speech correction and clinical audiology. *Journal of Speech and Hearing Disorders, 21,* 1, 5–11.

Cornett, B. S., & Chabon, S. S. (1988). *The clinical practice of speech–language pathology.* Columbus, OH: Merrill.

Culatta, R., & Goldberg, S. A. (1995). *Stuttering therapy: An integrated approach to theory and practicum.* Needham Heights, MA: Allyn & Bacon.

Dobson, K. S., & Block, L. (1988). Historical and philosophical bases of the cognitive–behavioral therapies. In K. S. Dobson (Ed.), *Handbook of cognitive–behavioral therapies.* New York: Guilford.

Fitts, P. M. (1962). Factors in complex skill learning. In R. Glass (Ed.), *Training research and education.* Pittsburgh: University of Pittsburgh Press.

Garber, J., & Seligman, M. E. P. (1980). *Human helplessness: Theory and applications.* New York: Academic Press.

Hegde, M. N. (1993). *Treatment procedures in communication disorders* (2nd ed.). Austin, TX: PRO-ED.

Holland, J. G., & Skinner, B. F. (1961). *The analysis of behavior: A program for self-instruction.* New York: McGraw-Hill.

Ingham, R. J. (1984). *Stuttering and behavior therapy: Current status and experimental foundations.* San Diego, CA: College-Hill.

Kazdin, A. E. (1980). *Behavior modification in applied settings* (Rev. ed.). Homewood, IL: Dorsey.

Klevans, O. R. (1988). Counseling strategies for communication disorders. *Seminars in Speech and Language, 9,* 3.

Kubler-Ross, E. (1969). *On death and dying*. London: Macmillan.

Lazarus, A. A. (1970). *Behavior therapy and beyond*. New York: McGraw-Hill.

Lefranqois, G. R. (1972). *Psychological theories of human learning: Kongor's report*. Monterey, CA: Brooks/Cole.

Leith, W. R. (1979). The shaping group: Habituating new behaviors in the stutterer. In N. J. Lass (Ed.), *Speech and language: Advances in basic research and practice*, (Vol. 2.). New York: Academic.

Leith, W. R. (1982). The shaping group: A group therapy procedure for the speech/language pathologist. *Communicative Disorders, 7, 8*, 103–115.

Leith, W. R. (1984). *Handbook of stuttering therapy for the school clinician*. San Diego, CA: College-Hill.

Leith, W. R. (2000). Communication disorders. In C. L. Radnitz (Ed.), *Cognitive behavior therapy for persons with disabilities*. Northvale, NJ: Aronson.

Leith, W. R., McNiece, E. M., & Fusilier, B. B. (1989). *Handbook of supervision: A cognitive behavioral system*. Austin, TX: PRO-ED.

Manning, W. H. (2001). *Clinical decision making in fluency disorders* (2nd ed.). Calgary, Canada: Singular.

Martin, G., & Pear, J. (1983). *Behavior modification: What it is and how to do it*. Englewood Cliffs, NJ: Prentice Hall.

Meichenbaum, D. H. (1993). Changing conceptions of cognitive behavior modification: Retrospect and prospect. *Journal of Consulting and Clinical Psychology, 61*, 202–204.

Meichenbaum, D. H. (1977). *Cognitive behavior therapy: An integrative approach*. New York: Plenum.

Meichenbaum, D. H. & Cameron, R. (1973). Training schizophrenics to talk to themselves. *Behavior Therapy, 4*, 515–535.

Mower, D. E. (1972). Accountability and speech therapy in the public schools. *Asha, 14*, 111–115.

Mower, D. E. (1988). *Methods of modifying speech behaviors*. Prospect Heights, IL: Waveland Press.

Mower, D. E., & Case, J. L. (1982). *Clinical management of speech disorders*. Rockville, MD: Aspen.

Othmer, E. O., & Othmer, S. C. (1989). *The clinical interview: Using DSM–III–R*. Washington, DC: American Psychiatric Press.

Post, J. (1983, April). I'd rather tell a story than be one. *Asha*, pp. 23–26.

Rokeach, M. (1980). *Beliefs, attitudes and values*. Washington, DC: Jossey-Bass.

Radnitz, C. L. (2000). A cognitive–behavioral approach. In C. L. Radnitz (Ed.), *Cognitive-behavioral therapy for persons with disabilities*. Northvale, NJ: Aronson.

St. Louis, K. O., & Myers, F. L. (1997). Management of cluttering and related fluency disorders. In R. F. Curlee & G. M. Siegel (Eds.), *Nature and treatment of stuttering: New directions*. Needham Heights, MA: Allyn & Bacon.

Seligman, M. E. P. (1975). *Helplessness: On depression, development, and death*. San Francisco: W. H. Freeman.

Skinner, B. F. (1974). *About behaviorism*. New York: Vintage.

Stone, J. R., & Olswang, L. B. (1989, June–July). The hidden challenge in counseling. *Asha*, pp. 27–31.

Van Riper, C. (1957). Symptomatic therapy for stuttering. In L. E. Travis (Ed.), *Handbook of speech pathology*. Englewood Cliffs, NJ: Prentice Hall

Van Riper, C. (1973). *The treatment of stuttering*. Englewood Cliffs, NJ: Prentice Hall

Van Riper, C. (1982). *The nature of stuttering*. Englewood Cliffs, NJ: Prentice Hall.

Watterson, B. (1988). *Something under the bed is drooling*. New York: Andrews and McMeel.

World Health Organization. (1980). *International classification of impairments, disabilities and handicaps: A manual of classification relating to the consequences of disease*. Geneva, Switzerland: Author.

Yaruss, J. S. (1988). Describing the consequences of disorders: Stuttering and the international classification of impairments, disabilities, and handicaps. *Journal of Speech, Language, and Hearing Research, 41*, 249–257.

INDEX

About the Author

William R. Leith is an emeritus professor of audiology and speech pathology at Wayne State University in Detroit, Michigan. He received his undergraduate degree from Western Michigan University and his master's and doctoral degrees from Purdue University. He has been a professor, teacher, speech pathologist, cognitive behavior therapist, consultant, author, and researcher at the University of Wichita, Colorado State University, Case Western Reserve University, and Wayne State University. He has maintained a private practice in stuttering therapy since 1975 in Cleveland, Ohio, and since 1980 in Detroit, Michigan. He has given lectures in 23 states, published over 50 articles, written five books, written four chapters for edited books, and made several professional videotapes for training clinicians, as well as holding numerous workshops throughout the country.

His books include *Clinical Methods in Communication Disorders (Third Edition)*, *Handbook of Stuttering Therapy for the School Clinician*, *Handbook of Voice Therapy for the School Clinician*, and *Handbook of Supervision: A Cognitive Behavioral System*. His unique clinical innovations have included The Shaping Group, a unique form of group therapy; Cognitive Behavior Therapy as applied to therapy for stuttering, voice disorders, and general communication disorders; Cognitive Behavior Therapy and clinical supervision; The Clinical Interaction Model: A Model in Therapy; Sensory Integration as applied to human communication; A training videotape for rating the severity of stuttering; and Systematic Desensitization with the telephone for stutterers.

He has received several honors for his contributions to the field of speech–language pathology, including being appointed a Fellow in and receiving a Certificate of Appreciation from the American Speech-Language-Hearing Association. He also received an honorary doctorate in speech pathology from Oulu University in Oulu, Finland.